W9-CRH-243

The Diabetes Question and Answer Book

Books by June Biermann and Barbara Toohey

Alice in Womanland
Cross-Country Skiing for the Fun of It
The Diabetes Question and Answer Book
Dr. Owl's Problem
From Baedeker to Worse
How to Ski Just a Little Bit
The Peripatetic Diabetic

The Diabetes
Question and Answer Book

_____

June Biermann and Barbara Toohey

Copyright © 1974 by June Biermann and Barbara Toohey. All rights reserved including the right to reproduce in whole or in part in any form. Address all inquiries to: Rights and Permissions Dept., Sherbourne Press, Inc., 8063 Beverly Blvd., Los Angeles, CA 90048.

ISBN 0-8202-0162-6
FOURTH PRINTING, 1976
Composition: Omega Repro, Tarzana, Calif.

To the diabetics who asked the questions and inspired us to find the answers.

Contents

Preface   i

FOR ALL DIABETICS

Why did I get diabetes?   3
What is diabetes?   3
Who gets diabetes?   4
Will I have diabetes the rest of my life?   5
How can I keep from being depressed over my diabetes?   5
Which is the correct thing to say, "I am a diabetic" or
    "I have diabetes"?   6
Will diabetes shorten my life?   7
Will my diabetes give me any sex problems?   8
How come I didn't have any symptoms of diabetes
    when my case was diagnosed?   9
Since I'm just a borderline case, will anything happen
    if I ignore my diabetes?   10
How can I find a doctor who specializes in diabetes?   10
How often should I see my doctor?   11
Why does my doctor always examine my eyes so
    carefully?   11
Will diabetes make me blind?   12
Why do I need to know so much about diabetes? Why
    can't my doctor take care of everything, if I go to
    him regularly?   12
How can I learn how to take care of my diabetes?   13
Is it really possible to live a normal life with diabetes?   15

What is a remission?   17

What are the chances that we'll have a cure for diabetes
    soon?   18

How can I find out about new discoveries in diabetes?   19

Should I tell people I have diabetes?   20

Can I have children and, if I can, will they have
    diabetes?   23

Why is it that I can't make myself do what I should to
    control my diabetes?   24

Is there any way I can cut the cost of my diabetic
    supplies?   26

Will I have trouble getting insurance because of my
    diabetes?   26

What does it mean to be in control?   27

What is diabetic coma?   28

What is hypoglycemia?   28

Can a diabetic who doesn't take insulin or pills ever
    have low blood sugar?   29

What is ketoacidosis?   29

What is a brittle diabetic?   30

Is it true that taking pills to help control your diabetes
    is bad for you?   31

What should my blood sugar be?   32

What is spilling?   32

How often should I test my urine for sugar and
    ketones?   32

Can I ever stop testing my urine for sugar?   33

How come I spill sugar even when I don't eat?   33

What is the kidney threshold?   34

Is it true that diabetes gets worse when you have a cold
    or the flu or even just some little infection?   34

How much should I weigh?   35

Why do doctors always insist that diabetics give up
    smoking?   35

Why do they talk so much about diabetic foot care?   36

I've been told I shouldn't sit with my legs crossed. Is this true? 37

I have a bad case of acne. Could this be caused by my diabetes? 37

What happens if I cheat on my diet? 38

How can I make myself follow the diabetic diet? 38

What are carbohydrates? 39

Is there anything I can eat all I want of without counting it in my diet? 41

Can a diabetic follow a vegetarian diet? 41

What about health foods for diabetics? 42

Will vitamins help my diabetes? 43

What is the Food Exchange System? 45

Do I have to eat on the Food Exchange System? 46

If something isn't listed in the Food Exchange System, can I still eat it? 47

I hate milk. Do I still have to drink it on my diabetic diet? 49

Can I save up food exchanges from one meal and use them for the next? 49

Do I have to measure my food? 50

Why am I supposed to read the contents part of the label on all food products I buy? Aren't all brands more or less alike? 51

I've been told a diabetic shouldn't eat concentrated sweets. What are concentrated sweets? 52

Are artifical sweeteners all right for diabetics? 52

Are coffee and tea bad for a diabetic? 53

Why is it that I can eat a meal and not show any sugar afterwards and then eat the very same meal again and spill sugar? 54

How can I eat the diabetic diet without imposing it on my family? 54

What do I do for dessert in restaurants? There's almost never fresh or unsweetened fruit. 55

What things should I eat a lot of?   56

Can't I ever go on a splurge and have something wild
     that's not on my diet?   56

How can I stay on my diet when I'm invited out to
     dinner?   56

Can a diabetic drink alcohol?   57

Since some doctors let diabetics drink alcohol, why
     shouldn't they also let them smoke marijuana?
     After all, marijuana doesn't have calories or
     carbohydrates.   59

Does exercise keep you from gaining weight?   60

How often should I exercise?   61

What should I do if I'm always too tired to exercise?   61

What sports are good for a diabetic?   63

Are there any countries you consider particularly good
     for diabetics to travel in?   64

What shots should a diabetic take before traveling
     abroad?   66

Are there any special things a diabetic should take with
     him on a foreign trip?   67

Can I buy my diabetic supplies in foreign countries?   68

How can I avoid getting diarrhea when I travel in
     foreign countries?   69

Why do I spill so much sugar when I go on a long
     airplane or automobile trip?   70

How can I get special diabetic meals on airlines?   71

How can I eat in foreign restaurants without wrecking
     my diabetic diet?   73

FOR INSULIN-TAKERS

Why do I have to inject insulin with a needle? Why
     can't I just take it in a pill?   77

Why do my insulin injections sometimes hurt?   77

When should I take my insulin?   78

What if I forget to take my insulin injection? 78

Do insulin syringes and needles require a prescription? 79

I'm getting little hollow places in my thighs and wherever else I give my injection. Why is this happening and is there any way I can get rid of these hollows? 79

I'm always afraid of having an insulin reaction when I'm asleep. How can I make sure this doesn't happen? 80

I've been told I should keep a supply of glucagon on hand. What is glucagon and how is it used? 81

I'm troubled by false attacks of insulin shock. I think I have low blood sugar and I drink a Coke or something and then I spill sugar like mad. What can I do about this? 81

Is it O.K. to exercise alone if you take insulin? 82

How can I know exactly how much carbohydrate to eat to keep me going through a game of tennis? 82

Is it all right to drive a car alone on long trips? 83

How can I keep my insulin the right temperature when I travel? 83

What do I do about taking insulin when I'm traveling and change time zones? 85

FOR FRIENDS AND RELATIVES

My husband wants to think and talk about his diabetes all the time. How can I get him off the subject? 89

How can I tell if a diabetic has low blood sugar? 90

What should I do for a diabetic who has low blood sugar? 90

What should I do if I find a diabetic unconscious? 92

If my diabetic child goes to a birthday party or trick or treating on Halloween, is it all right for him to break his diet just this once? 93

Should I give up eating pastries so my diabetic husband
    won't feel tempted?   94
My father has diabetes. Is there any way I can keep
    from getting it?   95
How can I help my child accept his diabetes?   95
Should I give my husband his insulin injections?   96
If I mention my wife's diabetes in a restaurant to try
    to get her something special, like a substitute for
    sweet and sour pork in a Chinese dinner, she gets
    furious and says I make her feel like a freak. What
    can I do?   96
What should I do if we're out dining in a restaurant
    and my husband, who is diabetic, orders all the
    wrong things for himself?   97
My son wants to play football. Is that safe for a
    diabetic?   97
Should I hire a diabetic?   98
How do I plan a meal for my diabetic friend?   99
My little boy has had temper tantrums since his dia-
    betes was diagnosed. Is this normal?   102
My daughter is diabetic. How can I find out more
    about diabetes and how to help her?   102
Appendix A: Affiliate Association of the American
    Diabetes Association   107
Appendix B: Recommended Weight for Diabetics   117
Appendix C: Food Exchange Lists   121
Appendix D: Daily Menu Guides   133
Appendix E: Some Convenience Food Equivalents   143
Appendix F: USV Ethnic Diets   151
Appendix G: Special Ethnic Exchange List of the
    Diabetes Association of Southern California   171
Appendix H: Chart of the More Common Foreign
    Equivalents for Oral Drugs Sold in the United
    States   181
Appendix I: Counting Carbohydrates in Foreign
    Countries   185

Appendix J: Some Helpful Tips on Filling Your Insulin
    Syringe   189
Appendix K: Two Accepted Techniques for
    Self-Injection   197
Appendix L: What Foods Can Be Served on Diabetic
    Diets   201

Preface

EVERY DIABETIC HAS something besides his disease, and that something is a head full of questions about diabetes and how to live with it. We know, because the June half of our writing collaboration is a diabetic. When her disease was diagnosed, she had so many questions that she would have needed a doctor and a dietician living with her twenty-four hours a day to answer them all. Now, seven years later, we finally have most of the answers.

Since, besides being writers, we are both college librarians, we tried to find the answers to June's questions in books. No luck. It turned out that there was not one book that gave answers to the most important questions we had, those about how to *enjoy* life as a diabetic. As a result, we had to learn everything the hard way, bit by bit and step by step and mistake by mistake. After a long period of research and experiment and hundreds of diabetic adventures, we took all our material and wrote a guidebook to good health and good times for diabetics, *The Peripatetic Diabetic.*

After our book was published, we were frequently invited to speak to diabetes associations. In the question and answer period that followed these talks there was always a lively exchange of information. Since almost every group we spoke to had a doctor and a dietician in attendance for professional consultation, we often came away with as many answers as we gave. Much of what we learned at these meetings came from fellow-diabetics who shared with us their experiences and their original solutions to diabetic problems.

Now we have collected between the covers of this book the most important and most common questions diabetics ask. And we offer you honest, practical answers to these questions. For the most part, these answers are not flat, rigid, one-way statements of Ultimate Truth. They are flexible answers that open the door to many different possibilities. What we give you here, rather than rules, are guidelines which you can use to chart your own course in this most uniquely personal of diseases.

What we hope you'll gain from reading this book are the three vital ingredients to diabetic success: acceptance, knowledge, and optimism. We've learned from experience that with these three you can live a full, exciting, and happy life—in spite of your diabetes.

Questions for All Diabetics

Why did I get diabetes?

You certainly didn't catch diabetes from anyone, because it is not contagious. You did inherit it, because it is hereditary.

The way we've heard it explained is that heredity loads the gun, but something else has to pull the trigger. That something else is some form of stress. Probably one or more of these body stresses shot off your diabetes gun:

Overweight
> This is the major trigger-puller. Eighty percent of adult diabetics are overweight when diagnosed.

Aging
> Most newly diagnosed diabetics are over forty and, if you have the inherited tendency, your chances of getting diabetes are greater with each decade of life.

Physical trauma
> Surgery, an auto accident, a major illness—all of these can bring on diabetes.

Certain medications
> Cortisone has been known to trigger diabetes.

Pregnancy
> The additional demands on the body during pregnancy can bring on diabetes. Pregnancy—actually a miscarriage—led to Mary Tyler Moore's diagnosis of diabetes.

Emotional stress
> Emotional tensions or crises can induce diabetes.

What is diabetes?

Diabetes mellitus is the medical name. *Diabetes* means *water siphon* and *mellitus* means *sweet.* The early Roman diagnosticians called it the sweet water siphon disease, because the person who had it urinated a great deal and his urine tasted sweet. Yes, *tasted* sweet. In those days, tasting the urine was the only way doctors had of testing it for sugar. (And the doctors of today won't even make house calls!)

For years doctors thought diabetes was simply a lack of

insulin. They thought it was strictly a pancreas problem, since it is the pancreas that produces the insulin the body needs. Now, they're not so sure about this theory, especially when diabetes develops later in life. Some experts think that enough insulin is produced, but for some inexplicable reason it cannot get into the cells. There is some kind of blockage. Another recent theory is that diabetes is not a pancreas disease at all, but a blood vessel disease in which the first thing that happens is the thickening of the walls of the smallest blood vessels, the capillaries.

Whatever the fundamental cause of diabetes, we can be certain of one thing. When investigators finally do figure out exactly how diabetes works, they'll be a lot closer to devising a cure.

Incidentally, the correct pronunciation of diabetes is die-uh-BEET-ease, not die-u-BEET-us.

Who gets diabetes?

People in any continent or country, of any age, race, or sex get diabetes. Even dogs get it. We know a dachshund that's on twenty-five units of insulin.

In spite of its universality, diabetes does favor certain groups. The most likely candidates are those who are over forty, overweight, and related to diabetics. Seventy-five percent of newly diagnosed diabetics are over forty; 80 percent are overweight. Not only does diabetes favor the older, the fatter, and family members, it also is sexist. It prefers women; in fact, it prefers married women. And to get even more specific, it particularly likes to choose overweight women over forty who have given birth to a baby that weighed over nine pounds.

Besides being sexist, diabetes is inclined to be racist. In the United States, it favors black women. Their death rate from diabetes is the highest of any group—27 per 100,000 people as compared to 15 per 100,000 for white males, for instance.

The fact that diabetes is related to diet also influences who gets it. According to a 1964-65 study by the U. S. Public Health Service, about 45 percent of the diagnosed diabetics come from families with an annual income below $4,000. We presume this group has a high carbohydrate diet, because carbohydrates are the cheapest kind of food, and a high carbohydrate diet causes diabetes to develop sooner than it might otherwise.

Will I have diabetes the rest of my life?

Yes, unless a cure is discovered.

How can I keep from being depressed over my diabetes?

It's only normal to be depressed over having diabetes, especially when it's first diagnosed. All the cheerful remarks about how much nicer it is to have diabetes than leprosy or than being run over by a moving van, or some such nonsense, do no good at all. You know that it's *not* better than having nothing wrong with you.

You get the "why me?" reaction. "Why should *I* be selected to get this chronic disease?" "Why should *I* have to give up all my pleasures?" "Why should *I* be threatened with blindness or an early death, if I don't follow a rigid regime?" Why, indeed? There's really no reason. It's just the breaks of the genetic game. As a doctor told us once at a meeting, "Every person carries around about forty-four genetic defects." One of yours happens to be diabetes, and the fact is that some people draw out worse tickets than diabetes in the genetic lottery.

We found that when June, in fits of depression, was ticking off all the pleasures she'd have to give up because of diabetes, what she was really ticking off were habits rather than pleasures. Something like eating sweet desserts was a habit that she considered a pleasure, merely because she'd done it so often that it was comforting. The trick is to establish new *good* habits and turn them by constant use into pleasures.

It's not as hard as you may think. Eating a delectable,

juicy piece of fresh fruit can as easily become a habit-pleasure as eating a big, gloppy dessert. For many people a daily bike ride or after-dinner walk is a pleasurable habit, and it can be for you, too.

Furthermore, when you're thinking of the things you have to give up because of diabetes, think of these: you have to give up ever waking up with a hangover, either of the cigarette or alcohol variety; you have to give up discovering on a shopping trip that you've ballooned another dress or suit size; and you have to give up feeling like a sluggish blob because of lack of exercise. Now, those aren't such depressing losses, are they?

Finally, try to keep in mind that it's the human condition to be depressed from time to time. With your diabetes you've got a jim-dandy depression catchall. There is a natural tendency for you to lay your every woe on diabetes' doorstep. That's unfair to diabetes. Bad though it may be, it's not enough of a villain to be responsible for every dismal moment in your life. Even if you didn't have diabetes, you wouldn't be frisking around in a constant state of ecstacy. Or if you were, you might have a defect of far more serious consequences than diabetes.

Which is the correct thing to say, "I am a diabetic" or "I have diabetes"?

Either is correct. It doesn't matter how you say it, just as long as you *do* say it. It's a matter of personal preference. *Diabetes in the News* ran a reader survey to see which way most diabetics like it better. "I am a diabetic" won a clear victory. Most people thought it was more straightforward and more accepting of your condition.

A case can be made, however, for "I have diabetes." It sounds more as if you are giving yourself primary importance and your disease only secondary importance.

Either of these phrases will make you easily understood. Don't shy away from them and use something cryptic the way June did once on a flight to Hawaii, when she was trying to get her meal from the stewardess. "I'm on insulin," she said. "Could you serve me first?" The answer was negative. The problem, we figured out later, was that the stewardess, who was Danish, didn't have any idea what June was talking about. In fact, she probably thought that insulin was the name of some kind of group tour of the islands and that June was just trying to get a special privilege for no good reason.

When Barbara trotted back a few minutes later and made eyeball-to-eyeball contact with the stewardess and announced, "My friend is a di-a-bet-ic and she needs to eat. Could you serve her now?" the meal appeared a few seconds faster than immediately.

In the use of the words diabetes and diabetic, experts have very definite ideas about correctness. They don't like you to use diabetic as an adjective, unless what you're talking about actually has diabetes. For example, "The diabetic man had a diabetic dog," is all right, because both the man and the dog are diabetics. "The diabetic education lecture was held at the diabetic study center," is all wrong, because neither the education lecture nor the study center has diabetes. It should be, "The diabetes education lecture was held at the diabetes study center."

You wouldn't say "a diabetic specialist," unless the specialist you're talking about has diabetes. If he's a specialist in diabetes, he should be called a diabetes specialist. If he's a specialist in diabetes who has diabetes, then presumably he'd be referred to as a "diabetic diabetes specialist." But maybe you think this is being linguistically nit-picky. Maybe we think so, too; since, as you may notice, we often use the word *diabetic* in the unaccepted way.

Will diabetes shorten my life?

Theoretically, probably yes. Actually, probably no.

The classic estimate is that, all things being equal, diabetes shortens a person's life by one-third. Frankly, we distrust this figure as outmoded and too drastic for an in-control diabetic. But just for the sake of argument, let's accept it. What, then, does "all things being equal" mean?

Our interpretation is that if you do not have diabetes and yet you live the way diabetics do—you eat a perfectly balanced diet low in fats and sugar; you drink little or no alcohol; you do not smoke; you keep your weight slightly below normal; you get regular daily exercise and regular nightly sleep—then you will live one-third longer than a diabetic doing the same thing.

But let's face it. Without the incentive of diabetes to make them follow such an optimum life style, 99 people out of 100 won't do it. No, better make that 999,999 out of 1,000,000 won't do it.

Now, let's say all things aren't equal. You don't have diabetes. You are overeating—and eating all the wrong things—overdrinking, oversmoking, and carousing around and never exercising, except possibly in occasional violent week-end spurts. Will this shorten your life? Yes, very likely more than diabetes will.

So maybe it's true that diabetes takes away years; but diabetes, if it makes you lead a healthy life, also gives those years back again—and maybe several more, to boot.

Diabetes has another couple of dividends. During the years you do live, you feel better. And if your vanity bump is as highly developed as most of ours are, it may comfort you to know that the diabetic regime also makes you look a heckuva lot younger and more vital than the average way of life does. You are bright of eye, glossy of mane, clear of skin, and lean of body.

Will my diabetes give me any sex problems?

Uncared-for diabetes can cause sex problems. One of the symptoms that has been known to send undiagnosed diabetics (especially males) sprinting to the doctor in the first place is a diminished sex drive or impotence. Often, as soon as the diabetes is stabilized, the sex difficulty disappears.

Occasionally, there is also the problem that you may develop hangups about sex if you have hangups about your diabetes. As one psychologist put it, sex is 95 percent above the neck. If up there in your head you're stewing and fretting about how your diabetes is going to mess up your normal activities, your normal activities are likely to get messed up, and this includes sex. Some men have found themselves suddenly impotent for a while after their diabetes was diagnosed. Obviously, an above-the-neck problem. Many of these same men found that the problem disappeared as soon as they got back in control emotionally as well as diabetically.

In advanced stages of uncared-for diabetes, there can be loss of nerve function to the pelvic organs, resulting in physical rather than psychological impotency. In his column in *Diabetes in the News,* Dr. Donnell Etzwiler said, "Daily proper control and management of diabetes is the most important factor in minimizing the risk of this complication." It's hard to think of a better reason for sticking to your diabetic regime.

How come I didn't have any symptoms of diabetes when my case was diagnosed?

You were one of the thousands of hidden diabetics—people who have diabetes and don't realize it, because it's not advanced enough for noticeable symptoms. You're one of the smart ones. You caught diabetes early by a urine or blood sugar test before it had done any real damage.

If you neglect your diabetes in the future, that's when you will experience the classic symptoms of more advanced diabetes: excessive urination and thirst, increased appetite, loss of weight, slow healing of cuts, itching skin, easy tiring and drowsiness and, possibly, change in vision. But since you're one of the smart ones, you probably won't neglect your disease and won't ever experience these symptoms.

Since I'm just a borderline case, will anything happen if I ignore my diabetes?

Sorry to have to tell you this, but you *aren't* a borderline case. There ain't no such animal. As we were told at the Loma Linda Diabetes Education Program, being a diabetic is like being pregnant. You either are or you aren't. You can't be borderline pregnant and you can't have borderline diabetes. The old master of diabetes education, Dr. Elliot Joslin, says that if you ignore your diabetes ". . . the mild case neglected always gets severe."

Actually, the so-called borderline diabetics are the most likely candidates for arrival at the hospital in diabetic coma, since they are the ones most likely to ignore their disease until it demands attention.

A person with a mild case of diabetes needs to be just as regular about his testing, about seeing his doctor, and as careful about his diet as someone on sixty units of insulin. Maybe even more so. After all, if you're careful, maybe you'll never have to be on sixty units of insulin.

How can I find a doctor who specializes in diabetes?

Telephone your local diabetes association. They have a list of all the diabetologists (that's the official term) in your area. If your town doesn't have a diabetes association, then contact one in the major city nearest you. Contact the American Diabetes Association, 18 East 48th Street, New York, N.Y. 10017, telephone 212-752-8550, for this information.

You can also check your public library for a copy of *The Directory of Medical Technologists.* This book lists the specialists in all fields of medicine by state and city and tells their education and experience.

Your local hospital is another source of referrals.

If you have diabetic friends, you can ask one of them the name of his doctor. This method isn't too reliable, though, because your friend may be going to his doctor for some reason other than his expertise in diabetes. (Perhaps he's his golfing buddy.)

But however you go about it, it's definitely worth the effort to check around and locate a doctor who is knowledgeable and experienced in diabetes. We've discovered that the more a doctor knows about diabetes, the less rigid he is and the more willing to adapt the treatment to your particular life style. He's more interested in and less fearful of letting you try new approaches to see if they work for you.

How often should I see my doctor?

Regularly—whatever that means to you. June thinks it means every other month, because this is the schedule her doctor recommends for his diabetic patients. Certainly, few diabetics, mild or severe, could go too far wrong seeing their doctors and having a blood sugar test this regularly. Your doctor, of course, may have somewhat different requirements for you.

We probably don't need to add that if you are out of control and/or spilling ketones (see page 29), you would talk to your doctor without delay and not wait for the next regularly scheduled visit. In fact, if you develop a health problem of any kind, whether related to diabetes or not, you would check with your doctor about that specific problem, even if you had just been into his office the day before for a routine appointment and blood sugar test.

Why does my doctor always examine my eyes so carefully?

He's looking for changes in your blood vessels. The retina, located at the back of the eyeball, is the one place in the human body where doctors can actually see and inspect the condition of the blood vessels. No weakness in the walls of the retina blood vessels—bulging or hemorrhages—is good news, since these blood vessels reflect the condition of the vessels throughout the body. You see, eyes are not just the mirror of the soul as the poets say, but the mirror of the body as well.

Also, especially for diabetics of long standing, doctors are checking for evidence of diabetic retinopathy. In this extremely serious eye complication, tiny blood vessels multiply and burst, creating blind spots. Recently, however, treatment with laser beams has improved the chances of slowing down this complication of diabetes. And the best thing about this laser treatment is that it isn't a one-shot affair. If retinopathy develops again later—and it usually doesn't—you can have laser treatments again, up to 600 times, in fact.

Will diabetes make me blind?

The National Society for the Prevention of Blindness reports that diabetes is the cause of 11 percent of the legally blind people in this country. This makes diabetes the third leading cause of blindness. (Senile cataract and glaucoma are the first and second leading causes.) These statistics, the latest available, are from the last decade and do not reflect the improved treatment during the 1970s of the most serious diabetic eye problem, retinopathy.

Admittedly, these are frightening statistics; but remember, eye problems, like other serious complications of diabetes, generally do not develop in diabetics who maintain good control of their blood sugar. One patient at Loma Linda has had diabetes for sixty-four years and still has eyes in perfect condition.

The answer to the question is no, your diabetes will probably not make you blind, but you can make yourself blind by not controlling your diabetes.

Why do I need to know so much about diabetes? Why can't my doctor take care of everything, if I go to him regularly?

Diabetes is the great do-it-yourself disease. The only way your doctor can be totally responsible for you is to be inside your skin and live your life with you. We all know that's impossible.

As a matter of fact, you help your doctor as much as he helps you—or you should. Unless you give him accurate reports from your testing for sugar in your urine and valid information on how your diet is working, he is severely handicapped, if not totally defeated in his treatment of you.

Mabel Reynolds, head nurse of the Loma Linda Diabetes Education Program, summed it up well. "You are the chairman of your diabetic committee. No matter how expert the other members may be—doctors, nurses, dieticians, social workers, psychologists, well-informed family members and friends—if the chairman doesn't know what he's doing and keep control, the whole program falls apart."

How can I learn how to take care of my diabetes?

It's like learning about any complex subject. You take classes, read books, and join discussion groups. Fortunately, most diabetics now have the opportunity to do all these things. When June first entered the world of diabetes, there were only two well-known teaching centers in the United States—the Joslin Clinic in Boston and the Diabetes Detection and Education Center in Minneapolis—and both were well-removed from the West Coast. Most of the books were grim and outdated. Discussion groups there were, thanks to the local chapters of the American Diabetes Association.

Today there is an ample choice of teaching programs, and new ones are sprouting up almost every month, especially in California, which has become a veritable mecca for them. Most of these programs offer a one-week course in diabetic care; some are live-in, but most are for outpatients. It's our opinion, after having recently taken the course at Loma Linda University Medical Center near San Bernardino, California, that no diabetic should be turned loose to cope with himself without the benefit of classroom instruction of the type we received at Loma Linda.

Our course took one hour a day for five days. It was absolutely free and the class was small with lots of opportunity for student participation. It was taught by a team of four nurses, a doctor, a social worker, and a dietician. The schedule was as follows:

Monday—Diabetes: What Is It?
  Insulin and Oral Agents
Tuesday—Foot Care
  Emotional Adjustment
Wednesday—Meal Planning
Thursday—Meals for Special Occasions
  Coma and Hypoglycemia (Insulin Reaction)
Friday—Sick Day Rules
  Travel
  Late Complications

At the end of the five days we each received a beautifully designed certificate stating that we had completed the course, The Understanding And Care Of Diabetes, and it was signed by the director of the Loma Linda University Diabetes Center, Dr. Charles H. Brinegar, Jr.

Why can't we provide you with a complete and up-to-date list of teaching centers throughout the United States? Well, we requested such a list from the editor of *Diabetes in the News,* who answered: "I do not have an up-to-date list of diabetes education courses in this country. There are hundreds and hundreds—some ongoing, some short-term—and they change all the time."

What you have to do is contact your local American Diabetes Association affiliate and ask them for information about the teaching programs nearest your home (see Appendix A).

We think that one way of having an ideal vacation is to journey to some area not near your home where there is an outstanding diabetes education center—the Minneapolis Diabetes Education Center, the Joslin Clinic in Boston, the Utah Diabetes Education Center in Salt Lake City—and enjoy the tourist sights and activities in conjunction with attending classes. Loma Linda University Medical Center, for example, is near Palm Springs. That means golf or swimming or tennis in the morning, your diabetes classes in the afternoon, and dinner at night in one of the fine Palm Springs restaurants. A great vacation combination.

We suggest, also, that you join your local chapter of the American Diabetes Association. Meetings generally feature a guest speaker—a dietician, dentist, podiatrist, ophthalmologist, nurse, insurance agent. And, of course, there are all those other friendly diabetics to swap stories with.

Is it really possible to live a normal life with diabetes?

According to Mary Tyler Moore, it is possible. "It never occurs to me that my life is anything but full and normal, nor should it be for any other diabetic who is in close contact with his or her physician." And that statement is from a celebrity who admits to an emotionally difficult period of adjustment to diabetes.

Of course, Mary Tyler Moore's life is not exactly what any of us thinks of as normal. We doubt that she would be satisfied living a blah normal life of doing the normal, expected, humdrum things every hour of every day of every year. Actually, we feel it would be no problem at all for a diabetic to lead a so-called normal life. What we're interested in—and what Mary Tyler Moore *does*—is lead an abnormal life and get away with it. And we mean *abnormal* in the dictionary definition of the word: extremely or excessively large. A bigger-than-life kind of life, a swinging life. Isn't that the kind of life you, too, *really* want?

One of June's greatest horrors when her diabetes was discovered was that her extremely or excessively large life of world travel, gourmet dining, skiing—in short, her life of doing whatever wonderful thing she jolly well pleased—would be curtailed. And that, as a consequence, her writing career built around those subjects would be wiped out. For this reason, her orientation to diabetes has been one of keeping her life the beautiful, abnormal experience it has always been.

Happily, over the last seven years with luck and pluck and study and research while writing *The Peripatetic Diabetic,* plus lots of experimentation and a whole gang of mistakes, we're happy to report that June has found out how to keep on leading her abnormal life. And we now pass on our findings to you.

The secret is just two simple words: *strict control.* June is probably the most conscientious diabetic you'll ever meet. She tests her urine twice as often as the average diabetic normally does, at least five or six times a day. Her sleep regime is so rigid that the time schedule of the crack French National Railroad is sloppy and capricious by comparison.

June exercises as regularly as a Kentucky Derby winner. And she sees her doctor so often that she thinks people may be beginning to talk.

Now you may say that, although this kind of life sounds plenty abnormal, it doesn't sound like an "extremely or excessively large" and swinging life. But stay, we'll explain.

The urine testing June does isn't all that arduous. With the convenience of Tes-Tape and Diastix it is, in fact, a cinch. All this testing gives June a good idea of where she stands and lets her know when she should eat more to compensate for extra activity like skiing. The testing makes it possible for her to lead a much more physically active life than she could otherwise.

June's strict adherence to the diet does not mean that she eats only commonplace, normal foods. What it means is that she's gone to a lot of trouble to find out the content of the abnormal ones. June's still a gourmet diner. For example, a couple of years ago in Verona, Italy, one of our travel companions watched June stow away antipasto, cannelloni, and osso bucco and then asked with eyes as big as pizzas, *"That's* a diabetic diet?" It most definitely was.

June's sleep schedule is a rigid seven-hour one, because she likes it that way. She feels better with adequate sleep and she knows she looks better. (She's very vain.) Actually, diabetes gives June a beautiful, built-in, unarguable excuse to check out of a dull party early.

June considers the exercise a treat rather than a treatment. Not only does she enjoy skiing or golfing or bicycle riding, but she doesn't feel guilty about taking time out to do it. In fact, it makes her feel virtuous, because she's being so conscientious about getting the proper amount of exercise for her diabetic health.

Seeing her doctor more often than normal is also an advantage, because it allows her to ask questions about how far she can go in her attempts to lead this extremely or excessively large life she wants.

So you see, June is abnormally careful so that she can be abnormally free. Believe us, it's more than a fair exchange. It's a fantastic bargain, since it not only guarantees her a large life but a long one. And that's another thing June's after, because she's got an awful lot of abnormal living to do.

What is a remission?

A *remission* is a period when diabetes becomes less severe. For example, an insulin-taker might find that he can keep in control on less insulin or on diet and pills, or maybe even on diet alone. Or perhaps a pill-taker can get by on diet alone. Sometimes a remission lasts quite a while. Sometimes it is short-lived.

Particularly common is the remission that occurs in juvenile diabetes after insulin treatment begins. This often causes the parents, who are already desperately clutching at straws, to think their child has been miraculously cured or that the diagnosis of diabetes was incorrect. False hope. Diabetes is still there. A remission is *not* a cure and should never be treated as such.

What are the chances that we'll have a cure for diabetes soon?

Things are looking up, at least, financially. In 1921 Banting and Best had a $100 budget to pay for dogs and, as you know, out of their research came the greatest diabetes discovery of all, insulin.

In 1951 the budget for diabetes research was up to $49 thousand and in 1971, it reached $8 million. Even so, there hasn't been a major breakthrough in diabetes research in thirty years. We're overdue. It's time for something to happen—something big.

What are the researchers working on? Lots of things. For example:

1. An insulin that can be taken orally.
2. An artificial pancreas. They have one now, but it's too large. What they're aiming for is one about three inches in diameter, approximately the size of a heart pacemaker. That's a pretty small package to contain all the good things they need to put in it: a glucose sensor to report the blood sugar level, a laboratory to analyze the findings, a computer to calculate how much insulin is needed, a reservoir of insulin that can be released in the proper quantity into the bloodstream, a pump, and a power supply for the whole operation.

One researcher predicts that at least a part of the artificial pancreas, the glucose sensor, will be ready by mid-1975 and, using it with an external radio receiver, diabetics will be able to check their blood sugar level at any moment of the day or night.

3. Pancreas transplants. There are, as in heart transplants, the two problems of getting the necessary organ and keeping the body from rejecting it after it's transplanted.
4. Beta cell transplants. The beta cells are the part of the islets of Langerhans in the pancreas that produce insulin. During the first experiments with animals, these cells were implanted in different parts of their bodies with only short-term success. Lately, researchers have had longer-lived success by injecting these cells into the large vein that leads

into the liver. The cells then plant themselves in the liver and proceed to produce insulin. The difficulties still to be worked out with this method include the familiar problems of finding the cells to inject and rejection by the body after they're implanted. One way both of these problems may be solved is by growing beta cells in a culture rather than taking them from another animal of the same species. When they've solved it with animals, success with humans cannot be far behind.

5.   Genetic change. This is science fiction stuff, but it may be the ultimate solution to diabetes along with every other human genetic flaw. It is a theory that someday when all the mysteries of genetic structure are solved, some sort of gene vaccinations to correct genetic defects will be found.

Finally, there's always the pleasant possibility that a cure or new control of diabetes that no one's even thought of yet will be stumbled upon serendipitously.

In the meantime, don't give up hope. Don't give up keeping yourself in control. When the discovery is made, you'll want to be in good shape to use it. And don't give up contributing to and working for diabetes research. Eight and a half million dollars for diabetes research may sound like a lot of money, but compare it with the 1969 defense budget of $85 million and you'll see it's as small as a grain of sugar.

How can I find out about new discoveries in diabetes?

You can keep an eye out for the word *diabetes* in newspaper headlines. The latest medical discoveries are usually covered first by newspapers. You have to be careful, however, not to let yourself get overly excited at reports of great breakthroughs. Reporters have a tendency to inflate small news items into zepplin proportions. When they get through speculating over what happened to three white mice in a laboratory in New Jersey, you're apt to be left with the impression that diabetes is soon going to be as passé as the black plague and you'll start making plans to run out for a double pecan pie a la mode.

Better and more realistic sources of diabetes information are the publications designed expressly for diabetics. If you join a local diabetes association, you'll probably get a news-letter and also the *ADA Forecast,* which is included in your dues. If you subscribe to the *ADA Forecast* independently, it costs $3.00. (Send your money directly to the American Diabetes Association, 18 East 48th Street, New York, N.Y. 10017.) *Diabetes in the News* is an excellent bi-monthly newspaper distributed free of charge by Ames Laboratories, makers of Clinitest, Diastix, Keto-Diastix, and Acetest. (Write to *Diabetes in the News,* 3553 West Peterson Ave., Chicago, Illinois 60659.)

Should I tell people I have diabetes?

Yes, yes, a thousand times yes. You should tell everyone you have any kind of everyday dealings with—your barber or hairdresser, your butcher, your baker, your candlestick maker, your colleagues at work, your insurance agent, all your friends, even rather casual ones. And you should espe-cially tell anyone with whom you have any kind of medical or semi-medical dealings, such as your dentist or podiatrist or oculist.

There are several good reasons for confessing your dia-betes. In the first place, should you have an insulin reaction, a person who knows you have diabetes can help you out or, at least, will realize that whatever is happening may be related to your diabetes and will get you to someone who can help.

You are also much less likely to inadvertently offend people if they know you have diabetes. For example, if you get low blood sugar and suddenly turn into a galloping grouch or a sarcastic put-down artist, they may realize that it's because of your diabetes. Then, too, if you're eating at a friend's house and turn down a sugar-shot confection, the cook will know that you're not insulting her talents but just behaving yourself and following your diabetic diet.

Another reason for announcing your diabetes to the world is that you can help out your fellow-diabetics by educating nondiabetics as to what diabetes is. What we diabetics need is an "each one-teach one" program so that we can spread diabetes facts and wipe out some of those weird fictions that are floating around in the public mind; such as, "A diabetic can't eat sugar, but he can eat all the honey he wants, because honey is natural."

If you tell about your diabetes, you're also likely to gain a lot of diabetic friends. That is to say, a number of people you already know will come out of the closet and declare themselves when you confess your guilty secret.

When June was first diagnosed, she was such a babe-in-the-woods that she didn't know that a lot of people hid their diabetes, as if it were a social disease rather than a metabolic one. She just blurted it out to everyone. To her amazement, it turned out that she knew five diabetics when she thought she didn't know any.

Later, June went through a period of diabetic self-consciousness and started covering up. That didn't last long. Barbara was always on the job spreading the news loud and clear. Every time we flew in an airplane, for example, Barbara informed the stewardess of June's condition and announced to the person occupying the third seat in our row, "My friend here has diabetes. Before lunch is served, I'm going to be giving her an insulin shot. I hope it won't bother you, but if it does, you can look the other way."

That used to make June cringe, but now in thinking back on it, she admits it was a good idea. After all, who knows what our seatmate might have thought was going on with that needle? And if June should need a quick snack, the stewardess would be alerted and would supply it fast and without question. Also, it helped her accept the fact that she has diabetes and not develop any psychological hangups about it.

As part of your diabetic announcement program, you should definitely wear some sort of identification bracelet or medallion. This is a safeguard in case you are ever in an accident or have some sort of diabetic problem when you're away from those who know you. A particularly good identification is a Medic Alert bracelet. (It is available from Medic Alert Foundation, Turlock, California 95380.) Medic Alert is well known now, and ambulance attendants and doctors and nurses in emergency hospitals are on the lookout for their insignia. June wears her Medic Alert bracelet always, even when she's asleep.

Now, after advocating this policy of extreme honesty, we shall hedge a bit and admit there is one circumstance in which a diabetic should be tempted to lie his head off. That circumstance is applying for a job or promotion when it is known that the company follows a ridiculous policy of not hiring or promoting diabetics. We don't mean such jobs as airline pilot, in which your diabetes might endanger lives if you had an insulin reaction on the job. No, we mean a job like architectural drafting or teaching high school botany or selling stocks and bonds, something in which diabetes couldn't possibly interfere with either your efficiency or the safety of others.

A friend of ours told us that her husband, who has diabetes, ran into this problem when they were first married. He had just graduated from college as a chemical engineer. She was pregnant. They had no money. Jobs were in short supply and he was desperate. He heard of an opening with an engineering firm, and he knew they required a physical before hiring. He couldn't afford to take any chances on losing out on the job because of his diabetes, so he smuggled a little vial of his wife's urine into the examination with him. When he was asked to provide a specimen, he provided hers.

When he came home, his wife asked him how his scheme

worked. "Great," he said, "they didn't suspect a thing." Then his face clouded. "Say," he said, "what if they run some kind of test on that urine and it shows that I'm pregnant?"

They didn't and he got the job.

Incidentally, we checked with a workmen's compensation attorney (Barbara's husband) who said that even if you've held back information on your diabetes and are injured on the job and the injury has nothing to do with your being a diabetic, you'll still be covered by workmen's compensation insurance. In some states, however, if your injury is caused by your diabetes (for example, falling into machinery while in a diabetic coma) it might be hard for you to collect.

Can I have children and, if I can, will they have diabetes?

You certainly can have children. If you are a man there is no problem at all. A diabetic woman may have complications that will cause a more difficult than normal pregnancy and, hence, a more expensive one.

A doctor told us that when one of his female patients with diabetes plans to get married, he calls in her parents and the groom's parents. He asks, "Do you want to be grandparents? O.K., then, are you willing to help out with the medical expenses of the pregnancy?" The future grandparents always say yes, the doctor reported, and he added with a smile, "I always hold them to their word."

Whether or not your children will have diabetes is a little harder to say. Although the diabetic inheritance pattern is not fully understood yet, the theory is that it works in much the same way as inheriting blue eyes or blond hair or some other recessive trait. If both parents have diabetes, it's virtually certain that all their children will inherit the tendency. If only one parent has diabetes, it's hard to predict how many, if any, of the children will inherit the tendency to the disease. It depends on whether the nondiabetic parent carries diabetes in his or her genetic make-up, too. You see, diabetes is never one parent's fault. Just as it takes two to tango, it takes two diabetes carriers to make a diabetic child.

We remember one mother of a diabetic child who said that she refused to send her son to a diabetes summer camp, because she was afraid he would fall in love with a diabetic girl and marry her, and they would have all diabetic children. The doctor who heard this story tried to put her mind at ease. "After all," he said, "a fellow doesn't fall in love with a girl just because they have diabetes in common. And besides, I don't think you need to worry about this summer, since your son is only ten years old."

Incidentally, we've read that because diabetics are now living so long and reproducing so well, some scientists are predicting that in a few centuries everybody will have diabetes. By then, if we're lucky, we'll probably have a cure for it.

Why is it that I can't make myself do what I should to control my diabetes?

It's probably not, as you may secretly think, that you're weak and wishy-washy. Most of the time, when a diabetic resists taking good care of his diabetes, there are many and varied psychological reasons behind his resistance.

The most common of these reasons is refusing to accept the fact that you have diabetes. You deny your diabetes by behaving as if you don't have it. This is self-defeating. Not only will such a denial not make your diabetes go away, but it will make your diabetes worse—and may even make *you* go away.

What you need most of all is a heart and mind and gut acceptance of the fact that you are a diabetic and always will be. There is nothing harder to come by than this total acceptance. But it's well worth working for, because once you've achieved acceptance, all the other ingredients of a successful life as a diabetic come easily. In pursuit of acceptance many diabetics need the A. A. serenity prayer as much or more than do alcoholics:

> God grant us serenity to accept the things we can not change, courage to change the things we can, and wisdom to know the difference.

It also could be that you're angry about having diabetes and you're fighting it by not following its dictates, by not letting it run your life. This kind of fighting, however, is only fighting yourself. You're the only one who's going to get hurt. If you can use that anger constructively to defeat your disease and use that fighting spirit to fight for perfect control, you're sure to be a winner in every sense of the word.

Maybe your problem is an underdeveloped ego. Maybe you think, "What difference does it make if I live or die? I might just as well forget about diabetes and do what I please." If this is so, what you need to develop is a healthy feeling of self-esteem. Your attitude should be, "I'm such a keen kid the world needs me, and I'd better take good care of myself so I'll be around for a long time." Admittedly, developing this kind of attitude is one of life's big psychological problems for everybody, diabetic or not, and no one can spell out exactly how to do it.

These are just three of the dozens of possibilities. Solving your diabetes misbehavior problem may take a whole lot of time and thought and talk. Talk is important. A social worker told us that talking it out with someone close and understanding can sometimes work miracles. You may be amazed to hear the solution to your problem coming out of your own mouth. If you don't have someone you feel you can talk to in this way, then by all means get some help from a professional—a social worker, a psychologist, or a psychiatrist.

It's worth working on this problem with all your forces and resources, because, remember, you're such a keen kid the world needs you.

Is there any way I can cut the cost of my diabetic supplies?

By using the tactics of competitive consumerism—shopping around for the lowest prices—you can cut your expenses by as much as one-third. B-D disposable insulin syringes, for instance, range in price from ten cents to twenty cents apiece, depending on where you purchase them. In 1973, June paid as much as $2.49 and as little as $1.64 for an identical bottle of insulin at two different pharmacies.

Buying in quantity is also sometimes advantageous. You can strike a bargain with an independent pharmacist by saying, "What will the price be if I buy a hundred instead of twenty-five of those pills?" He may or may not give you a break.

Certain of the health insurance plans will foot part of your drug bills, but you have to file prescriptions and keep receipts and accurate records in order to collect from them. Generally, they will pay only a portion of your expenses and only prescription items. For needles and insulin you may have to have your doctor file a prescription directly with the health insurance company. Find out the rules of your particular plan, figure out what you are entitled to, and be aggressive about making your claims stick. Unless you're loud and persistent, some insurance companies often don't pay.

Will I have trouble getting insurance because of my diabetes?

You shouldn't, but if you find that an insurance company is giving you a hard time or trying to charge you an exorbitant rate, there is help available. Write to Digitus, 1069 Springfield Drive, Campbell, California 95125. Digitus is a referral service founded by a diabetic, Tom Sullivan, for diabetics who want to buy insurance. Digitus will put you in contact with firms that will insure diabetics and insure them at reasonable rates.

According to an article on insurance for diabetics in *Dia-*

betes in the News, the following companies are known to give diabetics a fair deal:

Diabetic Insurance Programs, Inc.
P.O. Box 72
Westport, Conn. 06880

Jon W. Hall & Assoc., Inc.
6550C Troost Avenue
Kansas City, Mo. 64131

Continental Casualty Company
Offices in all major cities. Offers weekly hospital cash plan, hospital-surgical plan, and income protection plan.

What does it mean to be in control?

When a diabetic says, "I am in control," he means that most of his urine tests are showing no sugar and, presumably, his blood sugar is staying normal or near normal. When he says, "I am out of control," he means his urine tests are regularly showing 2 percent or more sugar, and were he to have a blood sugar test he would score above 150 or 160 (see page 32).

Admittedly, there are different degrees of control. We've seen charts that give descriptions that allow you to rate your control as excellent, good, acceptable or poor. In his *Diabetes Manual,* Dr. Joslin says that to have control of your diabetes, you must have at least one sugarfree urine specimen each day. June's doctor defines control as having sugarfree urine at least two-thirds of the time.

Most doctors warn insulin-takers that trying to walk too narrow a line in maintaining control may subject them to too great a risk of insulin shock. This holds especially true for juvenile diabetics. One doctor suggested that about 25 percent of an insulin-dependent diabetic's urine tests should show sugar, but never the same time of day every day. (That would indicate a poor diet pattern or incorrect insulin dosage.)

What is diabetic coma?

What diabetic coma means is that your blood sugar is high—it may be well over 1000—and your sodium bicarbonate and carbon dioxide level is low. Oddly enough, you don't have to be unconscious to be in diabetic coma. Only 15 percent are.

To define it more bluntly, diabetic coma is what out-of-control diabetics die of. In 1970, 37,800 American diabetics died of diabetic coma, even though death from diabetic coma has been totally preventable since the discovery of insulin in 1922.

To avoid ever getting yourself into this dangerous state:

1. Never neglect testing your urine for sugar and, if there is a lot of sugar, for ketones, too.
2. Never neglect taking your insulin or pills.
3. Whenever you are ill, check with your doctor to see if you need to take more insulin or pills.
4. Always be sure you are eating enough carbohydrate; this means that you shouldn't try to control spilling (see page 32) by eating less carbohydrate than your diet specifies.

What is hypoglycemia?

Hypoglycemia is the medical term for low blood sugar. It is the condition diabetics get when they take too much insulin, eat too little carbohydrate, or exercise too much.

Besides meaning low blood sugar, hypoglycemia refers to an ailment which is more or less the exact opposite of diabetes. In this disease the person's pancreas secretes too much insulin and he has symptoms similar to those of a diabetic with low blood sugar. Hypoglycemia, oddly enough, is sometimes a precursor of diabetes.

Can a diabetic who doesn't take insulin or pills ever have low blood sugar?

Indeed he can. Even nondiabetics can have low blood sugar. Anyone who exercises too much or eats too little or does both of these in combination can develop low blood sugar. The remedy is the same for everyone: eat or drink some carbohydrate.

KETON

What is ketoacidosis?

Ketoacidosis (or just *ketosis* or *acidosis*) is acid poisoning. It is what leads to diabetic coma and to death. It is brought on by lack of insulin. You probably know by now that insulin is like a key that unlocks the cells, so the sugar which the cells use for fuel can get in. When, because of a lack of insulin, not enough sugar can get into the cells, the liver produces ketones from the body's own fat and muscle to fuel the cells.

When ketones are burned as fuel, they give off an acid waste product which makes your blood become acid and you get ill in two ways: (1) you are literally eating yourself, consuming your own flesh and muscles, and (2) your cells are bathed in an acid solution.

The symptoms you experience are: frequent urination, thirst, headache, nausea, vomiting, abdominal pain, dim or blurred vision, and what is called *air hunger,* deep, slow, heavy breathing, along with a fruity-smelling breath. You become extremely weak, because the excess urination causes a loss of sodium and potassium. Others looking at you might notice that your skin appears dry and your face looks flushed.

Only a doctor can treat ketoacidosis and preferably in a hospital. Until the doctor arrives, you should go to bed, keep warm, and drink warm broth to replace your lost salt and potassium.

Ketoacidosis, you might be interested to know, leads to

death very quickly. Perhaps you remember reading about the California boy, Wesley Parker, whose father threw away his insulin because a faith healer had "cured" the boy's diabetes. Within three days, Wesley was dead.

What is a brittle diabetic?

The little glossary in the Ames Company's pamphlet, *Clinilog*, defines *brittle diabetes* as follows:

> Also called "fragile," "unstable," or "labile" diabetes. That type of diabetes in which the amount of sugar in the blood may change rapidly from too high to too low.

On the other hand, Dr. Leona V. Miller, chief of the Diabetes Section of the Los Angeles County/University of Southern California Medical Center, claims that there is no such thing as a brittle diabetic. We asked her to explain and she replied,

> Many physicians have used the term [brittle] in the past to describe the juvenile-type diabetic who easily became hypo or hyperglycemic. I do not care for the term; mainly, I suppose, because it is so overused by patients. It is a great out for many patients and an excuse for why they are so poorly controlled.

According to Dr. Miller, the real reasons for poor control are as follows:

1. Poor dietary habits—irregular meals, etc.
2. Irregular amounts of exercise
3. Inadequate or improper testing of urine
4. General lack of knowledge about diabetes
5. Inadequate or infrequent checks on blood sugar
6. Improper dosage of insulin
7. Erratic life style
8. Emotional stress

On hearing Dr. Miller's list, June immediately agreed that every time she is out of control, it's for one of those reasons.

We both feel that, for the most part, calling yourself a brittle diabetic is indeed an out, if not a cop-out. We keep running into adult diabetics at meetings who announce—almost, it seems, with pride—that they are brittle. They act as if the fates have decreed that they shall swing back and forth from high to low blood sugar forever and ever, amen, and there's nothing they can do about it. Frankly, like Dr. Miller, we doubt it. We think that, most of the time, these swing-high, swing-low types might be better described by some other term than brittle, although it might not be a term they would be so willing to apply to themselves.

Is it true that taking pills to help control your diabetes is bad for you?

In 1970, at the end of an eight-year study of diabetics on different treatments, researchers at the University Group Diabetes Program (UGDP) revealed that they had found more cardiovascular disease among diabetics taking oral hypo-glycemic pills (tolbutamine or Orinase) than among diabetics controlled by either diet alone or by diet and insulin. Immediately, the Food and Drug Administration warned doctors that the pills should be used only with diabetics who couldn't take insulin or who couldn't get along on diet alone.

Many doctors experienced in the treatment of diabetes questioned the conclusions of the UGDP study and objected strenuously to having their methods of treatment curtailed on the basis of a single study. This controversy has not yet been resolved. Some doctors continue to give their patients the pills; others do not.

What should you do? If we were you, we'd try exceptionally hard to make it on diet alone. Some diabetics use pills as a substitute for will power. For example, June once watched in horror as another diabetic slurped his way through a hot fudge sundae. When she shrieked at him, he just winked, popped a pill into his mouth, and said, "That'll take care of it."

If you can't make it on diet, then we'd think seriously

about deciding whether to stick with the pills or to go on insulin. Discuss the decision at length with your doctor and, by all means, keep an eye out for reports of further studies and conclusions on the oral hypoglycemic controversy.

What should my blood sugar be?

We're glad you asked that question. Every diabetic ought to find out what his blood sugar is whenever he goes to the doctor and has it taken. If the doctor doesn't inform you of his own accord, put the question to him and don't settle for an answer like, "It's normal" or "It's a little high." Demand to know the exact figure. He'll respect you for it. It shows you really want to understand diabetes.

Your blood sugar should be between 60 and 140. This is the normal range. If you can't remember this spread of figures, just keep in mind that it should be around 100.

What is spilling?

Spilling means that you have sugar in your urine. When the blood sugar goes above normal, the kidneys start spilling sugar into the urine. "I'm spilling," is the opposite of "I'm in control," because it means that you are out of control and have high blood sugar. The reason your doctor requires that you test your urine every day is to see if you are spilling. If you spill enough sugar for a long enough time, you will eventually end up in diabetic coma.

A believe-it-or-not fact: a wildly out-of-control diabetic can spill as much as two pounds of sugar in twenty-four hours.

How often should I test my urine for sugar and ketones?

The standard urine testing program calls for a urine sugar check before each meal and one before bedtime. That's four tests a day. For diabetics not on insulin and in good control, some doctors allow a reduction to one test either before breakfast or, sometimes, two hours after a meal.

Ketone tests are made only when urine sugar tests show three or four plusses on Tes-Tape (1 or 2 percent with Clinitest tablets). Some doctors recommend that patients with excellent control who never show more than a trace of sugar do an occasional ketone test just to keep in practice with the testing procedure.

Since urine and ketone tests are important information for your doctor as well as for you, it's smart to keep a written record of your tests. For this purpose the Ames Company has published an attractive, compact daily diary called *Clinilog,* which also contains a lot of valuable reference information. They'll send you a copy for $1.00. (Write to Dept. JRP, Ames Company, Division Miles Laboratories, Inc., Elkhart, Indiana 46514.)

Can I ever stop testing my urine for sugar?

Not unless you want to end up in a diabetic coma. In fact, the people who do get themselves into the hospital with coma are often the mild cases who stop testing, because they run negative tests for a year or so and get bored with the whole thing and give it up. After they stop testing, the next stop, a couple of years later, is the hospital.

How come I spill sugar even when I don't eat?

The liver releases sugar even when you're not eating. This is why when you're sick and have to cut down on your food, you can't skip your insulin or oral medication. In fact, you'll probably need additional medication, because the liver produces even more sugar during illness, and the body releases a hormone that makes insulin less effective.

What is the kidney threshold?

The *kidney threshold* (also known as the *renal threshold*) is the point at which your kidneys direct sugar into the urine instead of into the blood. The kidneys do this when the blood sugar is too high. The kidneys usually react in this way when the blood sugar is about 170 or 180—only about ten or twenty milligrams above normal blood sugar levels. If you have an average kidney threshold, you will find sugar in your urine whenever your blood sugar is over 170 or 180.

Some diabetics have a high kidney threshold. That is to say, the kidneys do not divert sugar into the urine until the blood sugar is over 180. The blood sugar may even have to be over 200 before sugar shows in the urine. For this reason a blood sugar test is the only truly accurate way of checking diabetic control and why you should have a blood sugar taken about every other month, especially if you think you might have a high kidney threshold.

One of our fellow librarians, who is, incidentally, a *fellow* librarian, almost never shows sugar on his Tes-Tape, unless he's been down in Baja California on a carbohydrous orgy of beer, beans and tortillas. Yet, when he goes in for his blood sugar tests, they usually are over 180, because of his high threshold.

Is it true that diabetes gets worse when you have a cold or the flu or even just some little infection?

Yes, it's true. This explains why diabetics controlled by diet or diet plus pills are sometimes put on insulin temporarily while they're ill. It explains why insulin-dependent diabetics, when ill, often have to increase their dosage or take regular (fast-acting) insulin before each meal in addition to their usual morning injection.

At Loma Linda University Medical Center, we were taught certain sick-day rules for diabetics to follow and we pass them on to you:

1. Continue whatever medication you take. Don't give up insulin or pills just because you don't feel like eating.
2. Test your urine more frequently than usual and test for ketones as well as sugar.
3. Call your doctor and report your condition and problems to him.
4. Drink broth (chicken, beef and vegetable are equally good), especially if you are vomiting. This will replace the sodium and potassium you are losing and prevent the dry heaves. Insulin-takers may also have to drink Coke, tea with sugar, or ginger ale to provide enough carbohydrate to avoid insulin reaction.

How much should I weigh?

A little less than you did in your early twenties. (If you're in your sixties, seventies, eighties, or nineties, still less than you weighed in your twenties.) At about the age of twenty-five most of us are at our ideal weight. A diabetic should keep slightly below his ideal weight in order not to overtax his ailing pancreas (see Appendix B).

A very simple and convenient test of the correctness of your weight is to pinch up your flesh just below your ribs at your waistline. Pressing the flesh between your thumb and forefinger, you should find a thickness of between one-half and one inch. If the pinch test reveals more flesh than that, you're too fat.

Why do doctors always insist that diabetics give up smoking?

Smoking is dangerous for everyone, but doubly dangerous for diabetics. Inhaling cigarette smoke affects the blood vessels. Diabetes affects the blood vessels. Both diabetes and smoking tend to narrow them, and narrowed arteries can cause heart disease and gangrene.

A diabetic has 2.5 times the normal chances of getting heart disease. A smoker has 1.7 times the normal chances of dying of heart disease. Put the two together and you'll have over four times the normal risk of heart disease.

A diabetic has sixty times the normal chances of getting gangrene of the feet. Again, smoking increases that already dismal figure. You might call smoking a form of Virginia roulette for diabetics.

So why are there diabetic smokers? We can't figure that one out.

Why do they talk so much about diabetic foot care?

It's that same old vascular story. Diabetes causes hardening and narrowing of the blood vessels. This, in turn, causes poor circulation of the blood. Since the feet are farthest away from that great blood pump, the heart, they get the worst deal. Poor blood circulation is also part of the aging process. So if you're elderly *and* diabetic, you've really got to watch those feet.

Here are the negatives:

1. Avoid crossing your legs.
2. Avoid elastic garters or anything tight around the legs or ankles.
3. Do not use heating pads or hot water bottles on your feet.
4. Avoid smoking; it reduces the blood supply to the feet.
5. Never walk around barefoot.
6. Do not use corn plasters or medications.
7. Do not cut corns or calluses.
8. Do not put your feet in water above eighty-five or ninety degrees.

Here are the positives:

9. Wash your feet every day and wear clean socks.
10. Always dry well between your toes.
11. Cut your toenails straight across.
12. Wear well-fitting shoes and change them frequently.
13. Examine your feet daily for signs of infection.
14. If you develop foot problems, go to a podiatrist (foot doctor) and tell him you are diabetic.

If it takes a horror story to make you behave yourself in the foot department, the Loma Linda Diabetes Education Program has a humdinger. It is about a man who didn't take care of his diabetes *or* his feet. As he aged and deteriorated, he lost his sight and all feeling in his feet. Well, it came to pass that one night, without knowing it, he knocked his watch off his bedside table and into his shoe. He walked around on said watch for two weeks. Needless to say, he wound up as a guest in the Loma Linda hospital. Incidentally, the average stay in a hospital for a diabetic with foot problems is twenty-eight days. Put that bill in your mailbox and see how much it takes to pay it off.

But the purpose of diabetic horror stories is not to scare you out of your wits. It's more to scare you into your wits. As Loma Linda's Dr. Brinegar put it, "We wouldn't tell you these things unless there was something you could do to avoid them."

I've been told I shouldn't sit with my legs crossed. Is this true?

It sounds like a bunch of old wives' nonsense and diabetic nit-picking, but there is some sense to it. Since diabetics are already prone to blood vessel narrowing and loss of flexibility, they shouldn't create even more blood circulation difficulties by throwing up crossed-leg roadblocks. Crossing your legs constricts the veins through which the blood is trying to fight its way back to the heart.

If you must cross something, cross your ankles. Or for even greater comfort and to give your circulation a hand instead of a handicap, buy yourself a footstool and prop those feet up when you read, watch television, or rest up after some extensive exercise.

I have a bad case of acne. Could this be caused by my diabetes?

Probably not. Many diabetics have a tendency to figure that every physical problem that appears is related to their diabetes. It is true that diabetes, especially out-of-control diabetes, is the great complicator, and it can whomp up a minor health problem into a not-so-minor one.

Still, you should try to avoid laying the blame for everything on diabetes. Not only does this make you feel more depressed and put upon, but it may also cause you to delay seeking treatment for whatever your problem really is—from acne to V.D.

What happens if I cheat on my diet?

If you do it once, you'll do it again and again and again. And each time you do it and run your blood sugar up, you risk damage to the body and the development of the serious complications of diabetes—heart disease and stroke, blindness, kidney and nerve damage, and gangrene of the feet.

The classic rationalizations are: "Once won't hurt," "I can get away with it," "It's Christmas," "I can't offend the hostess," "It's my birthday," and "I'll be conspicuous." Consider yourself in a worse predicament than an alcoholic. He has to be a total abstainer from alcohol. You have to be a semi-abstainer from food, half on and half off the wagon at all times. A very precarious perch.

There are, however, three exceptions when we think it is O.K. to go ahead and cheat on your diet. In fact, we heartily recommend it. These exceptions are: (1) your 100th birthday; (2) your golden wedding anniversary; and (3) your inaugural banquet, should you be elected president of the United States.

How can I make myself follow the diabetic diet?

You can conjure up horror stories in your imagination about the terrible things that will happen to you, if you don't. But a strong positive approach is better. Make your meals so delicious and interesting that you *want* to follow your diet. Make your eating not a grim therapy, but a pleasurable delight. Try new recipes. Try variations on old recipes. Try different herbs and spices. (Most of these are free, diabetically speaking.) And don't overlook the aesthetics of food serving. A few flowers on the table give you no extra carbohydrates or calories and do a lot toward making mealtime a pleasure.

This all holds especially true if you live alone. June, in her pre-diabetic days, often used to have for dinner what we called an avocado sandwich maybe; since whenever someone asked her what she was having for dinner, she usually responded vaguely, "Oh, I guess I'll have an avocado sandwich maybe," which meant she had no idea what she was going to have and didn't intend to make any plans. She was going to grab whatever she found in the refrigerator, if anything.

Now, June always has a well-planned, balanced, and delicious meal that she eagerly looks forward to. Her appetite is also better. Who knows if it's the better food or the limited servings that makes every morsel seem the more precious—but who cares? What matters is that she's eating less now and enjoying it more.

The most ghastly diabetic diet idea we've ever heard of is the result of a man's decision that calculating the diabetic diet is too much of a chore. He resolved to eat the same breakfast, the same lunch, and the same dinner every day. Ugh! Besides being lethally boring, this is nutritionally unsound. Diabetics need a lot of variety in their diets in order to make certain they're covering all the nutritional waterfronts. Not only that, but, as a home economist told us wryly, "You should eat a great variety of foods, because there are so many chemicals in everything these days, it's the only way you can avoid getting a big build-up of one chemical that might cause harmful side effects."

What are carbohydrates?

Not too many people recognize a carbohydrate when they see one. But, then, it's not easy to see the family resemblance between such different-appearing foods as oranges, potatoes, chocolate bars, corn flakes, and cabbages. The main connection in all these foods is a chemical one. They are all made up of carbon, hydrogen, and oxygen. And with the exception of the milk carbohydrate (lactose), they are all a part of plants. Another way to define carbohydrates is to say they are stored plant energy, and energy is exactly what they give the human body.

Carbohydrates are like the common man. God must love them, because he made so many of them. In the United States approximately half of our diet is foods that are mainly carbohydrates. In rice-eating Japan, 80 percent of the diet is carbohydrate. Carbohydrates are so much in evidence and so tempting that often to a diabetic the question seems more like, "What *isn't* a carbohydrate?"

The reason diabetics have to be so concerned about carbohydrates is that they are the kind of food most likely to cause sugar in a diabetic's urine. Some carbohydrates appear in the form of sugar (chocolate bars, soft drinks) and some in the form of starch (potatoes, corn flakes). It's important for diabetics to know that the sugars get into the blood faster than the starches. Starches have to be changed chemically by the body before they can become blood sugar, and that process takes time.

Also, not all sugars and starches have the same concentration of carbohydrate. White granulated sugar, for instance, is 99 percent carbohydrate. Apples are only 14 percent, and green beans a mere 7 percent. This explains why diabetics are allowed a lot of beans but virtually no white granulated sugar.

In the Food Exchange System (see page 45) of diabetic diet calculation, the following groups of foods are mainly carbohydrate:

Fruit exchange—10 grams
Vegetable A—5 grams
Vegetable B—7 grams
Bread exchange—15 grams
Milk exchange—12 grams

Fortunately for diabetics, carbohydrates are the most flexible of our food needs. You can reduce the amount you eat more safely than you can reduce any other dietary essential. In fact, if a person wants to reduce, eating less carbohydrate is one way to do it. (The carbohydrate which is not immediately used as fuel is deposited on the body as fat.) Most diets for diabetics contain less carbohydrate than the normal person eats. But even a diabetic can't do totally without carbohydrates in his diet. Not only are they the primary fuel food, but they also help the body utilize fats and protein.

Is there anything I can eat all I want of without counting it in my diet?

Yes, you can eat all the unsweetened rhubarb, unsweetened cranberries, and unflavored gelatin that you can possibly hold. Yum!

But seriously, folks, you can hype up the flavors of your meals with herbs and spices without counting them. And some dieticians hold to the theory that you can eat all of any vegetable A you want, as long as you eat it raw.

Can a diabetic follow a vegetarian diet?

It takes a pretty smart (excuse the expression) cookie to follow the standard diabetic diet. It takes a near genius to follow a vegetarian diabetic diet, especially if it is the strict vegetarian diet which eliminates dairy products, eggs, and fish, as well as meat.

The problem is getting sufficient complete protein on a vegetarian diet. Complete proteins are needed by the body to build and repair tissue. Animal proteins are complete proteins; they contain all the necessary amino acids of which complete protein is composed. Vegetable proteins generally are incomplete. You can, however, form complete proteins by combining two or more vegetables having the necessary amino acids. One example is the Italian pasta i fagiola, which combines macaroni and beans to make a complete protein.

Another example is a Mexican burrito, which combines a flour tortilla with beans.

But consider these two examples. Do you see the problem for diabetics? Right. Too much carbohydrate along with the protein. Still, it must be possible to follow a strict vegetarian diabetic diet. After all, there are diabetics among the Hindus who practice strict vegetarianism.

If the diet you have in mind to follow is one that eliminates only meat, poultry, and fish but allows milk, cheese, and eggs, then the problem is not nearly so difficult to solve. You just make up your meat exchanges with complete protein foods like eggs and cheese and combinations of these with vegetables containing protein. Our home economist friend says that if you make a dish with one-third complete protein and two-thirds incomplete, then the dish will be a complete protein.

There are many good books to help you out with the theory and practice of vegetarianism. Two of the best are *Diet for a Small Planet* by Frances Lappé (Ballantine, $3.95) and *Recipes for a Small Planet* by Ellen Ewald (Ballantine, $3.95).

An interesting sidelight to vegetarianism is the theory that a vegetarian diet causes you to be placid and loving. Recent studies revealed that an extremely warlike tribe in South America practices vegetarianism and that their eating habits may be the cause of their violence. The theory is that they're always running around with low blood sugar, because they don't eat enough slow-feeding-into-the-bloodstream protein. From this example, it's easy to see how a vegetarian diet might further complicate the already complex blood sugar balancing act of a diabetic.

What about health foods for diabetics?

If you mean granola, home-baked bread, yogurt, soy beans, sunflower seeds, wheat germ, alfalfa sprouts, and all that, great! The more different foods you eat, the better. Just make certain that you know the caloric, protein, fat, and carbohydrate content (or exchange equivalent) of whatever you eat and limit your portions so that you stay within your diet.

June adores health foods but finds she has to go very easy on them, because many of these foods are laced with concentrated sweets—honey, coconut, dried fruits, brown sugar— and many of them are overpotent in carbohydrate, fat, and calories. For instance, one-half cup of sunflower seeds is 280 calories, 26 grams of fat, and 10 grams of carbohydrate.

Most health breads are also heavier than ordinary bread. One slice will often equal almost two bread exchanges instead of one. You can check this out by weighing a slice. Bread is usually 50 percent carbohydrate, so a slice weighing 60 grams contains 30 grams of carbohydrate, or two bread exchanges.

A couple of words of warning about buying health foods. First, they tend to be terribly overpriced, and sometimes, rumor has it, those costly organically grown fruits and vegetables aren't grown in any special way at all. Second, when you're in a health food store making your purchases and happen to mention that you're a diabetic, you lay yourself wide open for a how-to-cure-it lecture from any health food nut within earshot. This happened once to June. "You don't *have* to have diabetes, you know," said the nut with more than a kernel of fanaticism shining in her eye. "It's all a matter of diet. We wouldn't have *any* of those diseases like diabetes and arthritis and cancer, if only people ate the right kind of foods; foods that haven't had all their vitamins and minerals cooked out or washed out with chemicals. Now let me tell you how you can cure your diabetes. . . ."

June suddenly remembered she was terribly late for an urgent appointment on the other side of town.

Will vitamins help my diabetes?

This question is as controversial as the question of whether vitamin pills do anybody any good. There are doctors who claim that the only thing vitamin supplements do for most people is give them expensive urine. There are doctors who have a go-ahead-and-take-them-if-you-like attitude. And there are doctors who counsel their patients to take vitamin and mineral supplements to insure that they aren't missing anything vital in their diet.

Personally, we both take vitamins and minerals regularly and copiously. We do this because, despite the assurances of the Food and Drug Administration and of the doctor-professor newspaper columnists, we believe that much American food is depleted of vital elements. We also think extra vitamins and minerals make us feel better. Whether or not that feeling comes from the head or the body, we can't say.

As for diabetics, in particular, needing vitamins; it is logical that even if a diabetic eats a perfectly balanced and varied diet, his meals are limited in quantity. If, for example, he is restricted to one-half glass of orange juice in the morning, it's a cinch he's not going to get as much vitamin C as the person who can glub down a full eight ounces of it. Consequently, even one vitamin C pill a day—say, 100 milligrams—brings him up to a better C level.

And the same holds true for the rest of the letters of the vitamin alphabet. As Dr. Joslin says, "To be on the safe side, there is no harm in taking one standard polyvitamin—a mixture of all vitamins—daily."

We're glad you asked, "Will vitamins help my diabetes?" and not "Will vitamins cure my diabetes?" We, too, have read in books of vitamin-lore fables of how diabetics were able to give up insulin injections entirely after loading up on vitamin supplements and health foods. Don't give yourself false hope. To paraphrase the James Bond title, diabetes is forever. At least, now it is. If you have surplus money, it's better to give it to diabetes research to develop a real cure and not to quacks who are pushing a false one.

What is the Food Exchange System?

The Food Exchange System for meal planning is a tremendous timesaver for diabetics or for anyone who wants to stay on a well-balanced, low-calorie diet. Before 1942 when the system was invented, diabetic dining was a real hassle, unless you happened to be a trained dietician or nutritionist.

The Food Exchange System divides all the kinds of foods available into seven categories or lists (see Appendix C). Your doctor decides how many calories you are going to be allowed each day—1200, 1500, 1800. Then you are given a printed sheet which includes the lists and which tells you how much food you can select each day from each category (see Appendix D). You are also told how the selections must be apportioned throughout the day. Your day's quota of food might be divided almost equally between breakfast, lunch, and dinner, though breakfast is generally somewhat smaller. Or you might be assigned certain snacks between meals.

The first list of the seven exchange lists is labelled *foods allowed as desired* (need not be measured). It includes seasonings, coffee, tea, and bouillon, as well as raw group A vegetables like lettuce, tomatoes, celery, asparagus. List two is *group B vegetables,* list three is *fruits,* list four is *breads,* list five is *meats,* list six is *fats,* and list seven is *milk.* There's an unnumbered list called *miscellaneous foods,* where you'll find such strange bedfellows as chili sauce and ice cream.

The lists have been ingeniously worked out so that one serving of a listed food, properly measured, provides approximately the same number of calories—and amount of carbohydrate, protein and fat—as any other serving on that list. For example, if your diet includes one fruit exchange for breakfast, you can choose any fruit from list three. Since not all fruits are the same in calories or anything else, the list tells you the exact amount of that particular fruit you can eat— and we mean the *exact* amount. One fruit exchange could be one-half cup of orange juice, one cup of strawberries, two

fresh figs, or one-quarter of a six-inch (in diameter) cantaloupe, just to give you an idea of some of the measurements.

You may be amazed at which foods fall into which groups.
The bread list includes potatoes, lima beans, corn, and spaghetti, as well as all the foods we generally think of as breads,
like muffins and crackers. Avocados, bacon, and nuts are
classified as fats, along with butter, margarine, mayonnaise,
and salad oil.

By the way, if you'd like to have extra exchange list diets
to distribute to your family members and friends, you can
get them by writing to Eli Lilly and Company, Indianapolis,
Indiana 46206.

After using the lists awhile, you find you learn them by
heart and don't have to constantly refer to your diet sheet.
That's when dining becomes a pleasure again.

Our only objection to the Food Exchange System is that
the lists are too short. They don't include all fruits, for
instance, or every kind of meat that's at the butcher's. Yet,
you *can* eat anything, just as long as you know which list it
fits on and how big the serving should be. The lists also
ignore all the modern convenience foods, like canned soups,
frozen dinners, and packaged muffins.

June got so frustrated with the lists that we searched
around until we found some expansions. Still not satisfied,
we got together with a college home economist and calcu-
lated the exchange list equivalents of many of the convenience foods. These expanded lists are found on pages 204-269
of *The Peripatetic Diabetic,* and we've come up with some
new ones (see Appendix E).

Do I have to eat on the Food Exchange System?

No, there is also a *free diet.* Frankly, though, we hate to
mention it, because all of us human beings being what we are,
are likely to say, "Whee, that's for me. I'll take that good old
freedom." Then, like one of those emerging nations that

suddenly gets its freedom, we may find we don't have the background to cope with it.

Still, we don't want to keep any secrets from you, so here's the free diet as described by Nancy Yeager, editor of *Diabetes in the News.*

> A free diet is one in which you do not have to weigh and measure foods, as long as you eat a basically nutritious diet that includes protein foods, milk products, fruits, vegetables, and cereals. The diet is not completely free because the amounts of sweets are usually more restricted.

Sounds great, doesn't it? There are, however, a pair of hazards here. First, you have to know exactly what a basically nutritious diet is. That's not easy. There is probably no other area in modern life in which otherwise intelligent, informed; and well-educated people are such utter boobs as in the area of nutrition. At the college where we work, you can take everything that our learned professors know about diet and fit it into the cap of a ball-point pen.

There is also that old devil problem of self-control. Without the guidelines of the Food Exchange System, there's a terrible temptation to increase the amounts of the things you like best and cut back on those that don't please your fancy. Immediately, your diet is thrown out of balance, and eating the wrong amounts of the right things is almost as bad as eating the right amounts of the wrong things.

We feel that using the exchange system is like having a car with automatic transmission. It's a lot less trouble than shifting for yourself and for most of us less than expert operators, it insures a smoother ride.

If something isn't listed in the Food Exchange System, can I still eat it?

Boy, can you! The exchange lists are often the first great shocker you get when your diabetes is diagnosed. From that

small collection of plain foods it looks as if you're con-
demned to the squarest parade of square meals ever thought
up by a dietician with dead taste buds. Not so. The exchange
lists are just a guide designed to simplify eating, not, as it
appears, to sentence you to a lifetime of meal boredom.

As we said before, in our *Peripatetic Diabetic* we published
greatly expanded exchange lists and even gave the exchange
equivalents of many quick-preparation foods, like Betty
Crocker mixes and Birds Eye frozen foods. We also included
a whole cookbook that shows how, still following the exchange lists to the letter (vegetable A, vegetable B, etc.) you
can eat sukiyaki or enchiladas or shish kebab or virtually any
exotic thing you want.

The clue here is knowledge of food values. This is what
sets you free from rigid eating patterns. Admittedly, acquir-
ing this knowledge takes some effort. June studied and
memorized Bowes and Church's *Food Values of Portions
Commonly Used* (Lippincott, 1966) as carefully as she would
have studied a foreign language she needed to conduct her
daily life in a foreign country. And it paid off. Now she can
eat almost anything and still adhere to her diet. If you do
likewise; you, too, can please virtually whatever gastronomic
fancy you may have. (Bowes and Church leave very little to
chance. They analyze such unlikely treats as reindeer milk
and raw racoon.)

Just about as good as Bowes and Church and a lot cheaper
($1.50) is the U. S. Department of Agriculture's Handbook
No. 8, *Composition of Foods, Raw, Processed, Prepared* by
Bernice Watt and Annabel Merril (revised 1963). For a copy
of this book write to the Superintendent of Documents,
Government Printing Office, Washington, D.C. 20402.

Almost any bookstore has two or three cookbooks for
diabetics, but they vary in kinds of recipes. We recommend
heavy browsing before purchase or, even better, seeing if
your public library can supply you with copies to try out
before you make the investment.

If you follow an ethnic diet, the USV Pharmaceutical Corporation (Tuckahoe, New York, 10707) has some exchange list guideline sheets for you. So far they've published a Jewish Diabetic Diet (in English and Hebrew), a Mexican-American Diet (in English and Spanish), an Italian-American Diabetic Diet (in English and Italian), and a Southern American Soul Diabetic Diet (see Appendix F). Also, the Diabetes Association of Southern California has made available through the courtesy of Pam Fulkerson, registered dietician at Northridge Hospital, special exchange lists for Latin American foods. These lists as well as her Chinese and Mexican menu exchange equivalents are included in Appendix G. For everybody, no matter what ethnic background, we've added her exchange list for McDonald's.

By putting a little time and thought into your meals you can make them just as interesting as they were before diabetes and maybe more so. But by all means don't let those exchange lists upset you. They are just a brief synopsis and, in no way, the whole story of your diabetic dining future.

I hate milk. Do I still have to drink it on my diabetic diet?

Good news! You don't. For each milk exchange you're supposed to be drinking, you can substitute one meat exchange worth of cheese and one fruit exchange worth of (what else?) fruit. This works out to about the same as milk in terms of carbohydrates, calories, and nutritional value. A lot of diabetics who love milk still make this switch once in a while for variety.

Don't forget that you can also use buttermilk and yogurt in place of milk.

Can I save up food exchanges from one meal and use them for the next?

Definitely not. One of the most important principles of the diabetic diet is having every meal well-balanced and eating neither more nor less than is called for. A diabetic, especially an insulin-dependent one, would really get into trouble if he tried to follow the great American eating pattern of nothing much for breakfast, a light lunch, and a gorging-session at night. As a matter of fact, all those non-diabetics who do follow this scheme are getting themselves into trouble, too. They don't feel their best, they don't function well, and they're putting on wads of fat.

The only exchange you can ever save up is your fat exchange. We don't mean that you can save fat exchanges for several days and then lap up a pint of whipping cream. It's more like saving one fat exchange from breakfast and one from lunch and using them at dinner. Even this shouldn't be a standard method of operating, only an occasional deviation.

Incidentally, you can get extra fat exchanges with every meal if you always drink nonfat milk. You get two—count them, two—extra fat exchanges for each nonfat milk exchange you drink. How's that for a deal?

Do I have to measure my food?

Yes. It's the only way to be sure you're getting the amount of food your diet specifies. It's not easy to recognize a half cup of orange juice or rice, unless you've measured them out a few times, and seven grams of beef would be even' harder. A gram scale is a good investment in the beginning of your diabetic days to get you on the right measuring track. After all, we're going to be switching over to the metric system pretty soon, anyway, and this will give you a head start. In a few years you'll be able to let the scale double as a postal scale.

At first, if you're really conscientious about weighing and measuring your food, you'll be amazed at how quickly you learn to eye-measure or, as with bread, hand-weigh, when you're out to dinner at a friend's house or in a restaurant. (Hint: sometimes it helps to discreetly nudge your food into little piles, the better to estimate the quantity.) You may get so good at this eye-measuring and hand-weighing that you can do weight and quantity-guessing parlor tricks, like the guy who guesses weights at the circus. Of course, the real and worthwhile trick is using your skill to eat the exact amount of food on your diet.

Why am I supposed to read the contents part of the label on all food products I buy? Aren't all brands more or less alike?

Brands are not only *not* alike; they are very different. Only by reading the fine print on the label can you know, for instance, whether a certain can of grapefruit juice contains sugar or not. Some brands do and some don't, and it's important for you to choose a brand that is unsweetened.

It's amazing how many food products have sugar thrown in. Fruits in heavy syrup are typical. You have to really search to find the few fruits, frozen or canned, that are unsweetened. Even cans of vegetables often contain sugar, as do canned meats, bottled salad dressings, frozen dinners, and endless other convenience foods.

Since the ban on cyclamates, there's even been a confusion with diet soft drinks. You have to realize that the term *artificially sweetened* does not necessarily mean without sugar. Drinks sweetened with saccharin often contain some sugar to counteract saccharin's bitter taste. On lo-cal drinks watch for the words *sugarless* and *sugarfree.*

As you read food ingredient lists on labels, you'll have to watch for the many chemical terms used to specify different kinds of sugars and starches. You should be aware that the following are all forms of carbohydrate: glucose, fructose, dextrose, sucrose, maltose, lactose, dextrin, and sorbitol—just to name a few.

Incidentally, ingredient lists are arranged according to the weight of each ingredient in descending order. The heaviest is listed first; the lightest, last. The lightest ingredients are usually those unintelligible chemical additives for which the American food processors have become famous. If you're baffled by what's going to be going into your stomach—and who wouldn't be with the likes of sodium metasilicate, calcium hydroxide, BHT, etc.—we suggest you read one of the current books which explains why these chemicals are in the foods we buy, what they do to it and to us. A few such titles we can mention to get you started are *200,000,000 Guinea Pigs* by John Fuller (Putnam, 1972), *Eater's Digest* by Michael Jacobson (Doubleday, 1972), and *Poisons in Your Food* by Ruth Winter (Crown, 1969).

I've been told a diabetic shouldn't eat concentrated sweets. What are concentrated sweets?

Concentrated sweets contain a high percentage of straight sugar. The straight sugars are white, powdered, brown or raw sugar, honey, molasses, and syrup. The higher the proportion of these in anything you eat, the more concentrated it is. Candy, jam and jelly, pie, syrup, cake, cookies, soft drinks— all the forbidden foods on diabetic diets—are exceedingly high in these sugars. They are taboo for diabetics, because they send the blood sugar soaring. So potent and fast-acting are these sweets that even nondiabetics can sometimes find small amounts of excess sugar spilled into their urine after eating a candy bar.

On the other hand, when sugar is used in small amounts and is diluted with other ingredients, as in bread, it feeds in more slowly. It gains a kind of innocence by association. It has neither the power nor the speed to send the blood sugar up rapidly.

Are artificial sweeteners all right for diabetics?

Well, they're better than downing an equal quantity of sugar. An occasional artificially sweetened drink is pleasant. We've found an especially good artificially sweetened tonic. Certain desserts like custard and gelatin and pudding would be pretty dismal without some sweetening and, if the sweetening is artificial, you can eat a more normal-size portion than if you were using sugar.

It's not, however, a good idea to load up on huge quantities of anything, especially anything chemical. You never know when it's going to dawn on the Food and Drug Administration that some chemical on their GRAS (generally recognized as safe) list has harmful side effects, as happened with cyclamates a few years back. One way to avoid getting too much of any one chemical is to buy several different brands of artificial sweeteners and alternate using them.

Much better than trying to fake a sweet taste with chemicals, however, is to lose your taste for sweets. If you're a sweet freak, this probably strikes you as utterly impossible. But the plain truth is that if you stop eating concentrated sweets, you eventually come to dislike them. Then, it is an affront to you if someone disguises the beautiful, natural flavor of a plate of strawberries by heaping it with sugar or several squirts of the artificial stuff.

Another good reason for not relying heavily on artificial sweeteners is that they help you, in effect, deny that you have diabetes. As we say again and again, acceptance is one of the most important factors in leading a successful and happy diabetic life.

Are coffee and tea bad for a diabetic?

Probably. Many recent studies show that drinks containing caffeine accelerate the aging process and cause heart trouble and genetic damage, and who knows what else? We've also read that caffeine has a tendency to artificially lower the blood sugar.

But, shucks, does a diabetic have to give up all his cherished habits? June drinks coffee. Sometimes if she feels she's starting to drink too much of it, she makes half regular and half decaffeinated coffee. She claims she can't distinguish a difference.

If you are a real addict, it would seem that you should cut

back or switch to decaffeinated coffee. (It would seem you should do this, even if you aren't a diabetic.) Certain conditions, like high blood pressure and insomnia, would also make eliminating caffeine advisable, if not imperative.

Why is it that I can eat a meal and not show any sugar afterwards and then eat the very same meal again and spill sugar?

This frustrating phenomenon happens to most diabetics. We've read that it can be explained by changes in the body's metabolism from day to day or, indeed, from hour to hour. Also, it stands to reason that variations in the amount of daily exercise, variations in the measurement of insulin and its absorption at different injection sites, as well as one's emotional state would influence what any specific meal does to the blood sugar.

How can I eat the diabetic diet without imposing it on my family?

What have you got against your family? Don't you want them to be healthy? Do you want to be the only one who feels well and looks good? Shame on you. You should *insist* that they follow the diabetic diet and eat well-balanced meals which include fresh fruits and vegetables and less refined sugar and fats. The diabetic diet is, after all, the perfect diet for everybody. We don't mean by this that everyone in the family will eat the same amount as the diabetic. If you have a strapping seventeen-year-old football player, he's going to need a heap more of calories to carry him throughout the day than you do. But he should get his calories from the same kinds of food you're eating.

It's not as if you are torturing your family. Diabetic meals, when prepared with imagination, are as good or better than those that would throw you off your diet. When June has guests, she always serves them diabetic meals. After stowing away the artichoke vinagrette, broiled salmon steak with horseradish, sherried carrots, homemade muffins, and fresh pineapple with mint, they look at her incredulously and say,

"*That* was a diabetic meal? I could happily eat diabetic meals the rest of my life." They could and they should.

You see, the ill wind of diabetes does blow some good. It turns the families of diabetics on to good eating habits. It may extend their lives as much as it extends the diabetics' lives. Barbara claims that June's diabetes is the best thing that ever happened to her, Barbara, in terms of decent nutrition. As she says, "If you really are what you eat, I used to be a greasy donut. Now, thanks to you, I'm more like a crunchy apple."

What do I do for dessert in restaurants? There's almost never fresh or unsweetened fruit.

You've just hit on one of the worst features of dining out in America. In Europe you virtually never have that problem. Fresh, delectable fruit is available in almost every restaurant, winter and summer. But here on home ground you're lucky if they can scare up a shriveled apple or dessicated orange.

You have a couple of choices of what to do. You can bring along your own fruit. You might get a few raised eyebrows now and then, but people's special dietary needs and preferences are getting more and more accepted. If you're shy about doing this, you can eat the fruit after you leave. June, when feeling a little low in blood sugar before a restaurant meal, has sometimes eaten her dessert fruit *before* going in. That way she can feel relaxed if there is one of those inevitable delays in being served.

Another alternative is to eat a scoop of ice cream. One-half cup of ice cream has just a few more carbohydrates and a whale of a lot more calories than fruit (160 compared to 40) and somewhat less nutritional value. Still, if you don't eat out regularly, missing your fruit once in a while isn't going to hurt.

One more point about fruit in restaurants. Don't give up. Always ask for fresh fruit for dessert every time you go to a restaurant, even every time you go to the same restaurant.

Eventually they may get the message. After all, there are around five million diabetics in this country and that makes us a pretty effective restaurant lobby, if we start speaking up for our rights as well as our apples, our grapes, our peaches, our pears.

What things should I eat a lot of?

Well, you shouldn't eat a gigantic lot of anything. One of the basic principles of the diabetic diet is great variety but small quantity. You could, however, say that, compared to the average American's diet, a diabetic should eat a lot of fruits and vegetables, especially the latter.

Can't I ever go on a splurge and have something wild that's not on my diet?

Yes, you can, and you have three choices about what you can do after the splurge:

1. You can spill like crazy and risk all the short and long-range problems that spilling causes.
2. You can go out immediately and work the splurge off with three violent sets of tennis or a five-mile run.
3. You can vomit it all up.

How can I stay on my diet when I'm invited out to dinner?

First, make sure that anyone who invites you to dinner knows you're a diabetic. That shouldn't be difficult, because if anyone knows you well enough to extend the invitation you will probably have long since told him about your diabetes.

Almost anyone who knows you're a diabetic will ask what's special about your diet. An easy way to explain it to them is to show them the answer to the question, "How do I plan a meal for my diabetic friend?" (See page 99.) If you don't have the book handy, just be sure to mention the piece of fruit for dessert. You might add that any vegetable is fine except succotash or corn and that potatoes aren't a vegetable to you, but rather they're like bread.

When you're actually eating dinner, do just as you would at home or in a restaurant. That is, don't eat more than you should just to be polite. It's always sound policy to wildly praise the hostess's cooking and express profound regret that you can't gobble up every morsel and even have second helpings. These words should work as well as lapping up everything to convince her that she's a wonderful cook. As a psychologist friend of ours says, "Cooking is a socially acceptable way of showing off." So long as the hostess gets the attention she's after, one way or the other, she'll be happy.

Incidentally, this was something of a sexist answer, implying that the cook is always a she. It's very possibly a man, in which case he's probably even more vain about his accomplishment and will need even more praise. Oops, that sounds still more sexist. We'd better sign off on this one.

Can a diabetic drink alcohol?

Here you have one of the great, if not *the* great, controversies about diabetes. Many doctors say absolutely no to alcohol. Not a drop. Others say it's all right in moderation. June has a joke which has some grain of truth in it. Question: "What did you do when your doctor said you couldn't drink?" Answer: "I changed doctors." There is some validity in changing doctors, if you insist on drinking and he insists that you don't. There is no point in going to a doctor if you intend to defy him or, even worse, sneak off and do something he forbids.

Actually, an excellent case can be made for a diabetic not to drink at all. Even alcoholic beverages that don't contain carbohydrate, such as gin, vodka, bourbon, scotch, and dry wines, do contain calories. Hard liquor of eighty proof has about seventy calories an ounce and dry wines have about seventy calories for three ounces. If you have any kind of weight problem, the additional calories of the drink will augment this problem. If you say, "O.K., I'll figure the calories of the drink in my diet and cut out something else," then that something else you cut out will have vitamins and minerals that alcohol lacks and your body will be deprived of them.

Then, too, drinking can get you in deep trouble, especially if you're an insulin-taker. Let's have a hypothetical story. Let's say it's the end of the day. Work is over. You're tired. You decide you'll have a pick-me-up drink before going home. You do. Then maybe you have another. Your judgment is suspended and your mind is a little fuzzy. You forget it's time for you to eat. In fact, it's past time.

You leave the bar and start walking several blocks to where your car is parked. Hypoglycemia comes over you. You stagger, stumble, and finally fall. You lose consciousness. Somebody calls the police to come pick up the drunk. The police arrive and, smelling alcohol on your breath, haul you off to the drunk tank to sober up. Very bad trouble.

Besides the dire possibilities of this scenario, there is also the possibility that the alcohol may throw off your medication or alter the effect of your insulin. Oral drugs combined with alcohol sometimes cause nausea and sweating. Alcohol may lower the blood sugar at the very time insulin is lowering it—just before a meal.

The case *for* drinking is weaker than the one against it but it is still there. For many people a glass of wine is a pleasurable adjunct to a meal. It is, in fact, for some national groups as much a part of the meal as the food. A small amount of alcohol is relaxing, and on festive occasions it makes you feel a part of the celebration. It would, for example, be sad not to have a glass of champagne at your own wedding. One glass of wine or a single mild drink makes you feel not nearly so left out and deprived as total abstaining does.

Even with your doctor's approval, however, before having a glass of anything you should do a little self-analysis of your drinking habits. Do you drink for the taste or for the effect? Are you the kind of person who can stop with one mild drink or one glass of wine? Or are you the kind who, once the first drink is down so are the barriers, and you have another, then another. If so, then don't take the first sip. There is no more lethal combination than diabetes and alcoholism.

Early on we developed a philosophy about diabetic drinking and with seven years of experience behind us it still holds. There are two reasons for a diabetic *not* to drink: the first is if alcohol means nothing to you and the second is if alcohol means everything to you.

Since some doctors let diabetics drink alcohol, why shouldn't they also let them smoke marijuana? After all, marijuana doesn't have calories or carbohydrates.

Even doctors who let their diabetic patients drink alcohol don't let them drink very much. They permit maybe one drink, enough to be sociable or to let the diabetic enjoy the aesthetic pleasure of a glass of wine with a meal. They never allow enough alcohol to mess up the diabetic's head.

When you smoke pot, though, no matter how bejewelled your roach clip, no matter how expensive an oriental carpet you recline upon, you're not smoking for sociability, nor for aesthetic pleasure. You're smoking for one reason and one reason only—to get stoned. And stoned is the last thing you need to be, especially if you're a juvenile diabetic on insulin. With your judgment impaired, you can easily forget to eat. You can forget to take your insulin or you might be unable to measure it correctly. All this can lead to one form of diabetic disaster or another.

Even non-insulin-takers can get themselves into trouble while seeking splendor in the grass. Following a diabetic regime is so complex that it demands all your faculties in good working order. You also have to consider the "munchies," that condition in which a marijuana smoker becomes ravenously hungry and wants to, and usually does, eat everything in sight. Think how that could louse up your diabetic diet.

Remember, too, that smoking pot is still smoking. *Playboy*

magazine once said that smoking, with its high cancer and heart attack odds, may be the big risk associated with marijuana use.

Finally, there are still a lot of unknowns about marijuana, more unknowns than knowns. Robert B. Forney, toxicologist at the University of Indiana Medical School, says, "We don't know nearly as much about marijuana as we know about cyclamates and birth control pills." As you may have noticed, most of the recent revelations about these two drugs have been bad news.

You already have one great complicator in your life— diabetes. Why compound the complication with a mystery drug like marijuana?

Does exercise keep you from gaining weight?

It certainly helps. Your weight is the result of how many calories you take in and how many you burn. If you eat more than you work or play off, then your weight goes up. If you use more calories than you take in, you lose weight.

The anti-exercise lobby has for years been trying to pass off the myth that exercise only works up a bigger appetite. They claim you eat more after exercise and not only don't lose weight, but even gain it. Lie! Our favorite nutrition expert, Dr. Jean Mayer of Harvard, has proven that those who exercise more actually tend to eat less than those who just sit around accumulating blubber.

Exercise also makes your metabolism more efficient and, if you're on insulin, makes your insulin work better. You get a double advantage from your exercise-induced calorie burning.

Another story the anti-exercisers like to tell is that it takes so much exercise to work off a pound of fat, it's futile to even try. Their favorite statistic is that you have to walk sixty-six and a half miles (at a rate of seventeen and a half minutes a mile) to lose one pound and, they ask, who can do that every day? Agreed. Probably nobody. But if you only take a fifteen-to-twenty-minute walk every day, it will add up to, or rather, reduce you by ten pounds a year. Take that, you anti-exercisers.

How often should I exercise?

Every day. Regularly. Exercise is basic to diabetic control. You shouldn't skip your exercise any more than you would skip taking your insulin or oral drug or skip eating.

We can't fathom why some diabetics resist the exercise part of their treatment. Exercise is the most pleasant part of the diabetic care program. And the nicest aspect of it is that diabetes gives you a keen excuse to indulge in exercise. A nondiabetic might feel guilty about dropping everything and going off for a bicycle ride or a round of golf or a swim or a long walk, but a diabetic can enjoy the exercise for itself *and* feel virtuous about doing it.

Besides participating in regular fun and games exercise, a diabetic can help his control and his health by just becoming a more active person: the kind of person who moves a lot instead of sitting a lot, the kind of person who uses stairs instead of elevators, the kind of person who prefers feet and bicycles to cars.

A story that brings home this idea of not compartmentalizing exercise away from daily life is one that was told to us about a friend's son. The boy is determined to be a tennis champion. He starts the day with calisthenics and a three-mile jog. Then when it's time to practice tennis, he asks his mother to drive him the eight blocks to the court.

What should I do if I'm always too tired to exercise?

To some extent, that depends on what you did to get tired. If you're weary from your job as steeplejack or long-shoreman, or if you're a housewife who's cleaned the whole house or galloped after a four-year-old all day, you've already had a great deal of exercise. Getting more is not that critical for you.

On the other hand, if you're tired from a long day of sedentary office tensions or sitting in the car, then you need exercise for more reasons than diabetic ones, and you should clamp your jaw and force yourself. Just as the appetite comes with the eating, the energy and enthusiasm for exercise come with the exercising. Often the fatigue you feel at the end of a day comes from a *lack* of physical activity rather than from too much of it.

Naturally, you'll be more likely to exercise, if you choose an activity you enjoy rather than one you detest. There are those of us, for example, who consider jogging a total bore. It's not bloody likely that we'd be able to stick to a daily dose of it for any length of time. We'd find excuse after excuse not to. So choose something you adore and do that. Or do several different activities you genuinely like. That's even less boring.

And speaking of varieties of exercises, there are two general categories: one that firms up muscles and redistributes weight (calisthenics, weight-lifting) and one, the aerobic variety, that builds up your cardiovascular system (walking, bike riding, jogging, tennis, skiing, swimming). For a diabetic the aerobic kind is by far the more essential exercise.

To find out what kind of aerobic shape you're in and how to improve it, you might look at Kenneth Cooper's book, *The New Aerobics* (Bantam Books, $1.25). There is also a splendid little pamphlet put out by the President's Council on Physical Fitness and Sports. It is called *An Introduction to Physical Fitness* and includes self-testing activities, graded exercises, and a jogging program. It can be obtained free by writing to the Council, Washington, D.C. 20201.

And one final word about exercise. If you find yourself too tired to exercise and it's not a true physical tiredness, you may go to bed and find yourself too keyed up and tense to sleep. The next day you've got a lack-of-sleep tiredness going. Vicious cycle. But if you get out there and move those bones around, blessed sleep will zonk you as soon as you hit the pillow. You'll sleep the sleep of the physically tired and virtuous. And you can't hardly sleep better sleep than that.

What sports are good for a diabetic?

Whatever sports the individual diabetic enjoys are good for him; these are the ones he's most likely to get out and do. That's the important part for a diabetic—getting out and doing.

If you've never been very enthusiastic about sports, then shop around until you find one that grabs you. Tennis is fine and fast and a lot of exercise. There have been diabetic champions like Bill Talbert and Ham Richardson. Golf is great, if you walk instead of using a cart. (One doctor claims that nobody should be allowed to use a golf cart without a medical prescription stating that he can't get around without one.)

Skiing is a little hazardous, but that shouldn't stop you, if you really like the sport. Studies show that the human animal needs to indulge in risk sports like skiing and horseback riding and mountain climbing, because they cause the same juices to be squirted into the system that squirted back in the days when we had to fight nature and beast for our primitive lives. The body functions better with occasional squirts of these juices. Also, sports like skiing keep you so scared that you forget about the fact that you even have diabetes.

Cross-country skiing is ideal for a diabetic for several reasons. You're less likely to break something than in down-hill skiing. The boots are light and flexible and less apt to cause diabetic foot problems, and it's great sport for building up your cardiovascular system. On top of all that, you do it out in beautiful natural surroundings, a great tonic for the spirit. We all know diabetes responds favorably to good spirits.

Ice skating is fine. Swimming is great. Bowling is O.K., except that you don't do it outdoors and there's a lot of eating and beer drinking associated with it.

There's nothing wrong with team sports, either, except that it's harder to dig up seventeen other guys for a baseball game than it is to get one guy for a few sets of tennis or a round of golf or a ski touring ramble through the woods.

And speaking of companionship, *always* take someone along, even if you're doing something you basically do alone like skiing or swimming. Even nondiabetics are advised, for safety's sake, not to do sports by themselves. For a diabetic it's twice as advisable.

Are there any countries you consider particularly good for diabetics to travel in?

Actually, a diabetic who does his pre-trip homework can travel happily in any country from Andorra to Zanzibar. After all, diabetics live in every country in the world. Why shouldn't other diabetics be able to travel there?

Still, there are certain countries where an American diabetic feels more comfortable than in others. There are countries where the food is more similar to our own and is more easily identifiable. There are countries where English is more commonly spoken and that makes diabetic coping easier.

Probably the best foreign country for a diabetic to start with in his travel experimenting is Canada. It's close. You don't have a grueling transoceanic flight. And it's foreign, yet familiar. French Canada is particularly good in this respect. You get the excitement of a different culture and yet you can get around easily, because everyone speaks English as well as French. The menus are usually printed in both languages, because bilingualism is a national policy.

After you've wet your diabetic feet with Canadian travel, then you should be ready to try Europe. The best countries, in our opinion, for a diabetic who's a bit nervous about foreign travel are: Britain, Ireland, Holland, Denmark, Norway, Sweden, and Switzerland. In all of these your English will get you around. The food is not too dissimilar from that which we find in our restaurants and, in all except England, it's usually a lot better. A diabetic, even one with comparatively little travel experience, can feel totally comfortable in these seven countries.

Our special favorite for diabetic travel is France, because there is no cuisine anywhere in the world that is better for a diabetic. Ah, the heavenly things they do to vegetables. Ah, the beauty of the fruit tray that appears at every meal. Ah, the perfect small-size portions. But aw, shucks, how those French do love to speak French and how they do love to read it on menus. So if you decide to go to France, especially outside of Paris, you should brush up on your French or pick up a little if you have none to brush up on.

In the mysterious East, we consider Japan the easiest place for diabetic coping. If you stay in Western-style hotels, there is always a Western-style restaurant, and very good it usually is, too. Even in the larger Japanese inns there are usually familiar things to dine upon. One of our most cherished memories of the Yama-No Inn near Lake Hakone is of the two of us in the dining room wearing the yukatas (Japanese robes) provided by the inn and devouring with our chopsticks a curry and rice dish, while all the Japanese in the room, wearing conservative business suits and dresses, were eating steak and potatoes and salad with knives and forks flashing.

The Japanese Travel Bureau does an excellent job of looking after Westerners, making sure they get familiar food and beds of the kind they're used to at home. Often they do such a good job that it's hard to convince them you really want to try doing things the Japanese way.

When you do have a Japanese dinner, two dishes to avoid are sukiyaki, which is loaded with sugar or mirin (a sweet wine), and miso soup, which is thick and risky. Go instead for the clear soup called suimono. And when you have a tempura dinner, don't forget to count the batter on the tempura and cut back on the rice accordingly.

Another possibility for diabetic ease and comfort in international travel—albeit an expensive one—is to stay only at large chain hotels, such as Hilton, Intercontinental, and Western International. In these hotels you can almost always get any kind of special diet you need or at least find familiar dishes on the menu.

Bon voyage.

What shots should a diabetic take before traveling abroad?

It's not so much what shots a diabetic should take as what shots anybody who doesn't want to get sick should take. Jerry Hulse, *Los Angeles Times* travel editor, says:

> Everybody knows by now that Uncle Sam welcomes you home without need of innoculations. Only if you've been to an infected area is it necessary to prove you've faced the needle. Still, as in the case with the driving permit, it is advisable to keep certain shots current. Besides smallpox, I continue to get boosters for tetanus, typhoid, and polio. Also, cholera and yellow fever if I'm entering an area where these two diseases are reportedly active. In addition, I received an injection a few days ago against hepatitis. I'm constantly accused of being a hypochondriac, but these are minor precautions against the possibility of major illnesses.

When we checked with our mutual doctor's nurse, she maintained that we didn't need a polio booster, because if you've had the sugar cube variety (one time when it's O.K. for a diabetic to have sugar), you're covered for life.

It's hard to decide about certain optional shots. A couple of them, namely cholera and typhoid, can lay a body low for two or three days. One doctor we talked to considers the tetanus innoculation the most important one of them all for protection against an accident.

A shot for which we have developed a particular fondness is gamma globulin. We were introduced to this one by a world-traveling woman who happens to be married to a doctor. This shot gives you short-term defenses against all manner of maladies and doesn't cause any kind of reaction; at least, we've never had any. Barbara, who used to fall victim to sore throats on European ski trips, hasn't had one since she started using gamma globulin.

Are there any special things a diabetic should take with him on a foreign trip?

Quite a few. Naturally, you take along all your regular diabetic supplies. Besides taking them along, be certain that they get there with you. Hand-carry them onto the plane in a flight bag, so they don't wind up in Bangkok when you wind up in Paris.

You will also need a generous supply of any other medication or vitamins you take regularly. And then there are the special medicines you may need for trip emergencies— Lomotil or something equivalent for diarrhea, an antibiotic, a decongestant, a bottle of regular insulin.

For a really long flight full of time-zone changes, we also take along a few sleeping pills. Since we never take them at home, they are tremendously effective. When your biological time clock is all mixed up, it's a comfort to be able to get eight solid restorative hours of sleep. Naturally, this you *must* discuss with your doctor and only take sleeping pills if he prescribes them, and then take them only for the first couple of nights, just long enough to get yourself into the new sleeping pattern. And a further caution. If you're an insulin-taker and are traveling alone, you'd better forget sleeping pills. A Nembutal combined with insulin shock would make a horrendous knockout drop.

In addition to the usual well-thought-out travel wardrobe, a diabetic should take at least two pairs of thoroughly broken-in walking shoes. It's astounding how much walking a tourist does and over what cobblestones and gravel paths, as well as sidewalks and asphalt. If possible, change your shoes a couple of times a day to make sure you aren't starting blisters anywhere.

A diabetic should carry a diabetic identification card in the languages of the countries to be visited. (Our book, *The*

Peripatetic Diabetic, includes samples.) Printed cards that ask where the restroom is are handy, too, when you don't know the language.

In case ot medical emergencies abroad, it's not a bad idea to join Intermedic, 777 Third Ave., New York, N.Y. 10017. This organization, for a small membership fee (under $10.00), will supply you with a list of 355 English-speaking doctors in 174 foreign cities along with a guarantee that they will treat you for a fair price.

June always carries a pocket flashlight so that she doesn't stub her diabetic toes in dark corridors on the way to the bathroom at night. (She's very considerate and doesn't turn on the light and wake up her traveling companion.)

We also carry a "carbohydrate arsenal" for those times when excess exercise wears down blood sugar or meals are delayed. This arsenal is made up of little packages of individually wrapped crackers, cookies, candy, pretzels, etc., which we've filched from baskets in restaurants or off the constant procession of airline meal and snack trays. June also always carries small plastic sandwich bags in her purse so she can make breakfast and lunch leftovers into small sandwiches for longer-lasting sustenance that may be needed during the daily sightseeing hike.

Another good thing to take along on your foreign travels is a friend or relative who understands your diabetes and you and can help you cope with the unexpected.

But probably the best thing to take with you, besides a thorough knowledge of diabetes, is a thorough knowledge of the customs and cuisine of the countries you're visiting. You acquire this information by reading a lot and questioning people who've been there before you. Fortified by this background, you feel almost as relaxed as if you'd been there before yourself.

Can I buy my diabetic supplies in foreign countries?

You can buy some of your diabetic supplies in all of the foreign countries and all of your diabetic supplies in some of the foreign countries, but you can't buy all of your diabetic supplies in all of the foreign countries. Given this mish-mash supply situation, the discreet diabetic definitely takes along everything he needs—oral drugs (see Appendix H), insulin, glucagon, needles, syringes, urine-testing materials, etc. In fact, to be on the safe side, it's a good idea to take along all you would need plus enough for one extra week. This way you are covered in case you decide you're having such a great time you'll stay longer, or in case you break or lose something en route, or in case you get stuck on a hijacked plane.

If you are a belt and suspenders type, as June is and as every smart diabetic should be; along with your oversupply of supplies, you will also take along prescriptions for all of your needs, even those that don't normally require a prescription at home. This way you'll be covered if all is lost—as it can be—and you'll also have some additional proof that you're a diabetic, should you have trouble getting needles across a foreign border. (In six years of traveling with needles, June has never been questioned at a border because of them.)

Taking your supplies with you is not just a safety precaution. It's a trip enjoyment insurance policy. On a foreign vacation, when there are so many glorious and exciting things to do and see, you definitely won't want to waste your time plodding from pharmacy to pharmacy trying to extract diabetes supplies from a pharmacist who may not understand what you want and who, even if he understands, may not stock what you're after.

How can I avoid getting diarrhea when I travel in foreign countries?

Sometimes you can't. Each country has its own varieties of bacteria in the water and food. The very fact that these are different from the ones you're accustomed to causes the well-known tourist trots. Their bacteria are not necessarily bad and ours good. They're simply different. That's why it works both ways. A Mexican who vacations in Chicago may get what might be called Sitting Bull's revenge, just as an American may get Montezuma's revenge while visiting Mexico City.

As a diabetic you should, of course, do everything you possibly can to protect yourself from diarrhea. In south-of-the-border countries where tourist trouble is a special threat, drink only bottled water and avoid drinks containing ice. Brush your teeth either in bottled water or in water that you've boiled. Don't worry about being accused of being a fussbudget. Just worry about not getting diarrhea.

When all preventive measures fail, you should take some kind of anti-diarrhea remedy. Naturally, you'll have to consult your doctor on this, but our favorite is a prescription drug called Lomotil. We like this for two reasons. First, it isn't full of carbohydrates like some of the anti-diarrhea clay compounds and, second, it's such a tiny little mite of a pill that you can swallow it with saliva, if you're not near a glass or bottled water and find yourself in distress.

Besides taking a remedy for diarrhea, you should try to drink a cup of broth every hour and have bananas as your fruit exchange. This restores the vital salts and potassium that are lost from your system during bouts of diarrhea.

Why do I spill so much sugar when I go on a long airplane or automobile trip?

A teenage diabetic basketball player who had to curtail his activities after minor surgery aptly summed it up. "I never realized how little you can eat when you're just sitting on your butt all day."

And sitting is what you're doing on an airplane or in a car. Consequently, either you have to cut back on your food or you're going to spill like crazy. An insulin-taker can increase his dosage slightly, *if* he's experienced at doing this and *if* he's not driving the car or flying the plane.

While we're on the subject, let us pause briefly for a tirade against the Great American Dream Vacation. You know, that's the one where you get up, have breakfast, drive for 250 miles, stop for lunch, drive for another 250 miles, check into a motel, have dinner, go to bed, sleep, and get up and start the whole dismal cycle again.

For a diabetic this is the worst possible vacation. In fact, for *anybody* it's pretty bad. In the first place, you're burning up a bunch of gas, a selfish and thoughtless thing to do in a time of energy crisis. In the second place, you don't really experience any of the places you visit—usually five-minute stops before you hustle back into the car so you can make your daily 500 miles. Third, it's no fun for anyone but the driver, because he's the only one who's doing anything at all. And how much fun is it even for him to hold onto a steering wheel and press with his right foot? And fourth, since nobody gets any exercise to speak of, everybody's likely to put on weight.

Far, far better to go to only one or two places and really enjoy them. Tramp all over the hills of San Francisco. Explore every byway of Taos. Go where there's a sport you enjoy, like golf or tennis or horseback riding or swimming, and really *do* it. Or camp out and hike and get acquainted with mother nature, who may not be around much longer to get acquainted with.

For your own sake, stay out of that car and stay off your you-know-what.

How can I get special diabetic meals on airlines?

You request them when you buy your ticket and the agent relays your order to the airline. If you change your flight number, you must inform the airline so that they can switch your meal order, too.

Which airlines offer special diet trays? Virtually all of them, foreign and domestic. Some have standard diabetic meals, while others ask that you specify exactly what you want and their catering service will prepare it for you.

The way the special meal service works is that you notify one of the stewardesses as you board the plane that they're carrying a special meal for you. If you don't identify yourself at the beginning of the flight, your chances of getting the meal are nil. Even if you do let the staff know, it's still pretty tough to get delivery. What happens is that the hurried and harried cabin staff forgets to serve you your meal or serves it last. (This can be a real problem for insulin-takers.) We've actually had stewards on international flights get angry over being reminded to deliver a special meal when they were rushing around trying to serve the starving hordes.

We've also found that the special diabetic meal is sometimes less appetizing and even less diabetically appropriate than the standard fare. One traveling diabetic friend reported, "You can't believe some of the things they serve diabetics on airlines." He particularly remembered the canned peaches in heavy, sweet (sugar sweet, not artificially sweet) syrup he got on one diabetic tray.

Frankly, we've tried the special meal a dozen or so times on about six different airlines and we've come to the conclusion that it's best to accept the regular airline meal. The regular meal is usually pretty well-balanced and includes some kind of salad and vegetable. The dessert, especially on domestic airlines, is often a sticky wad of carbohydrates, but that, too, can be fixed. After the cabin staff has served all the meals and starts to unclench their teeth and breathe normally again, you identify yourself as a diabetic and humbly supplicate for a piece of fruit for dessert. When we do this, the stewardess always sprints up to the first-class section and returns with a beautiful tray of perfectly ripe fruit.

By the way, we find that flying first class is a huge waste of money for a diabetic, unless you need it for leg room or for status. June can no more get her money's worth out of the parade of fancy foods and liquors and wines served there than she can at an eat-all-you-want pancake breakfast.

How can I eat in foreign restaurants without wrecking my diabetic diet?

It's often easier to eat in foreign restaurants than it is to eat in American restaurants. For one thing, in most foreign restaurants you can get fruit for dessert. For another, they usually do wonderful things with vegetables. (Never in a foreign restaurant have we seen that American restaurant horror, succotash.) Also, in foreign restaurants the meals are customarily served in small individual portions with several choices for each course. Except for pasta in Italy, you don't get the huge appalling mounds of food that American restaurants favor. In Scandinavian countries diabetics get a special break, because it's a cinch to select a perfect meal from the great variety of dishes on a smorgasbord or cold table, as it is called in Norway.

Every country, of course, has its national concoctions—its goulash, its boeuf bourguignonne, its paella, its cioppino. Unless you have a good idea of what's in these concoctions, you can get yourself into dietetic difficulties (see Appendix I). The way to solve this problem is to do a little homework before you take off. Get yourself a couple of cookbooks on the country you're going to visit and read up on the national dishes. Then you'll know what's likely to be in them.

If you get off the beaten tourist path and you don't read the language, you'll need a guide to foreign restaurant terms. We use Myra Waldo's *Dining Out in Any Language* (now out of print), but there are other good ones, such as Wilma George's *Eating in Eight Languages* (Stein and Day, 1968).

The red *Guides Michelin,* available for France, Germany, and Italy, offer menu terms and national cuisines in the front of each book, just as you would expect a guide published in France to do.

We've personally found that it's best to go to just one country or even just one major city, like Rome or Paris or

London, instead of doing one of the "If it's Tuesday it must be Belgium" hop-around tours. Staying longer in one place allows you to become really familiar and comfortable with one cuisine. It also gives you a chance to get out and walk and explore. That's better than loading yourself into a bus or train for a day-long ride. Even not figuring in your diabetes, it's the best way to travel. Instead of returning home with the whole of Europe as one vague blur in your mind, you really know Scotland or Madrid or the Austrian Alps or wherever you concentrated your travel.

Questions for Insulin-Takers

Why do I have to inject insulin with a needle? Why can't I just take it in a pill?

The digestive juices of the stomach destroy the insulin before it can be used. One of the goals of diabetes research is to develop an oral insulin that will work. Many scientists, however, consider this to be a more difficult feat than designing an artificial pancreas.

Why do my insulin injections sometimes hurt?

To have a painless injection you need a really sharp needle in the hands of a really sharp operator. A sharp operator drives the needle in like a dart hitting a dart board. Unless you do a quick, firm plunge with the needle, it won't sink in far enough, it may cause pain, and you'll probably have to start all over again. Nobody can give a perfect pop every time, but most of us can do it right most of the time. (For syringe-filling and injecting hints see Appendixes J and K.)

If you're hopelessly chicken or a constant botcher, there is a way out. You can buy an automatic pistol-like injector. You load a needle and syringe into the mechanism and just pull the trigger. Zap, the injection's over. There's also a very expensive compressed air gun called Hypospray, which sprays in the insulin. We've never received a response from the manufacturer (R.P. Scherer Corporation of Detroit) about the particulars of this mechanism. It's like ordering fruit in a restaurant: if enough of us keep trying, we may get some action.

As for the other half of the painless equation, sharp needles, there are as many as five or six brands in the disposable style. B-D (Becton-Dickinson), Jelco (Johnson and Johnson), Eisele, and Monoject are some of the more common names. Oddly enough, only B-D's are stocked by most pharmacies on the West Coast. Jelco's cannot be had at all or by special order only.

Our personal evaluation of the brands June has tried is that B-D's have easy-to-read syringes and not very sharp needles. Jelco's have superb needles and hard-to-read syringes. Eisele's have good needles, hard-to-read syringes and fall-apart sterility protectors. Monojects were recommended to us by the head diabetes education nurse at Loma Linda University Medical Center, but we've never been able to get our hands on one.

When should I take my insulin?

The answer to this question depends on how many injections you take a day. Most diabetics on insulin take one shot a day and that one is taken before breakfast; usually, the recommended time is one-half hour before eating. Other diabetics take two shots a day, one-half hour before breakfast and dinner. Still, a few others, and June is by personal choice one of these renegades, take one shot of regular insulin before each meal. These three shots are taken one-half to one hour before breakfast and almost immediately before the other two meals.

Of course, the actual daily timing of insulin injections cannot be all that precise, because life is so unpredictable. One morning you may oversleep, be in a hurry to get to work, and take your shot five minutes before breakfast. Another morning you may get an unexpected telephone call after the injection and delay breakfast for three-quarters of an hour. We've heard of even stranger variations from diabetics, like the man who told us, "Lots of times I eat breakfast and take my injection after I'm finished."

In the final analysis, each person has to work out his own best timing so that he can keep his blood sugar and his life style as close to normal as humanly possible. And then he has to accept the exceptions to his schedule with good grace.

What if I forget to take my insulin injection?

Congratulate yourself on not being obsessed with your disease. But if this happens more than just once in a blue moon, you'll need to devise some kind of a reminder system, like a nagging husband or wife. If you have a small child, you can give him a penny each time you take the shot. (He'll never forget.) When it does dawn on you that you forgot your shot, be sure to take an injection immediately—maybe less than usual, if you're well into the day.

Sometimes the problem is remembering whether or not you took the insulin. Then you have to worry about getting a double dose or no dose at all. A user of disposable needles can look into the wastebasket, if he empties the wastebasket every day. There's no doubt that a good memory is a help to a diabetic.

Do insulin syringes and needles require a prescription?

This one's a real puzzler. The answer is that they do and they don't. In California, for example, most pharmacists require only the diabetic's signature, but not the doctor's. Some, however, insist on a doctor's prescription. The laws vary from state to state and the interpretation of the laws varies from pharmacy to pharmacy.

We've never tried purchasing this equipment out-of-state, but June always carries a doctor's prescription in case the occasion should ever arise.

I'm getting little hollow places in my thighs and wherever else I give my injection. Why is this happening and is there any way I can get rid of these hollows?

What you have is called fat atrophy or, more scientifically, lipodystrophy. Insulin is what is making the fat disappear. Very few diabetics have this problem. Women, alas, are more prone to it than men and more prone to be disturbed by it when they get it. June has fat atrophy and we've asked every expert on diabetes we've come in contact with how to avoid it and how to get rid of it. No one so far has had an answer.

There are two items of hope, though. June stopped injecting in her thighs and other areas where she has fat atrophy and over a four-year period the hollows have been gradually filling in.

Also, when you start using U-100 insulin—and that should be any day now, if you haven't already—the risk of fat atrophy will be greatly diminished. You'll be injecting a much smaller volume of insulin and the insulin will have fewer impurities.

I'm always afraid of having an insulin reaction when I'm asleep. How can I make sure this doesn't happen?

If this is one of your worries, you'd better not read Bill Talbert's *Playing for Life*. He drinks too much one night, goes to bed without a snack, and wakes up in the hospital. The woman who rescues him from unconsciousness is now his wife.

We heard another somewhat unnerving story from the mother of a young diabetic boy. She had taken her son to Disneyland and let him enjoy himself to the hilt all day long. The next morning she couldn't awaken him, except with an injection of glucagon (see page 81). After he came to, he didn't feel well all morning, but he still wanted to go back to Disneyland again—and he did!

June's story is the opposite of these two horror tales. She finds that if she has low blood sugar while asleep, she wakes up with a feeling of nausea or some other telltale symptom. Then, it's merely a matter of grabbing the honey packet she keeps by her bedside or getting up and heading for the refrigerator. To avoid this kind of nocturnal disturbance—it's not unlike having to give a three-week-old baby his midnight feeding—it's a good idea to always have your prescribed snack before retiring and an extra-large snack, if you've had a lot of evening exercise or a slim meal at dinner.

And as a final word of comfort, in case your worry is really the ultimate fear that you will quietly die in your sleep, doctors unanimously agree that it's virtually impossible to die from an insulin reaction. Even without treatment the body is able to make a spontaneous recovery. (Doctors do warn, however, that insulin reactions are abnormally dangerous if you have heart disease.)

I've been told I should keep a supply of glucagon on hand. What is glucagon and how is it used?

Glucagon is a chemical that's injected in the same way as insulin, only it has the opposite effect of insulin. It raises the blood sugar. It's used to resuscitate diabetics who are unconscious because of low blood sugar.

Even if you never use it, glucagon is a nice security blanket. Just be sure whoever might be giving you an injection of glucagon knows where you keep it and how to administer it. And caution your family members or friends to inject glucagon when you're in insulin shock and unconscious, rather than trying to force liquid or food down your throat. An unconscious person cannot swallow and may choke to death.

I'm troubled by false attacks of insulin shock. I think I have low blood sugar and I drink a Coke or something and then I spill sugar like mad. What can I do about this?

Actually, you're doing the right thing already. If you have symptoms of low blood sugar, real or imagined, treat for low blood sugar. Better safe than sorry.

Occasional mistaken feelings of insulin reaction, we think, are bound to happen to every insulin-taker. But the first few years, while you're learning to judge your sensations, you'll do more misdiagnosing than after a period of experience. Sometimes you get a little twinge of a suspicious, though false, symptom and then fear takes over, giving you the sweats or dizziness or another convincing, but again false, symptom of hypoglycemia.

If you don't eventually outgrow or outwit this problem through self-education, then the only route left to you is to talk it out with a medical or psychiatric specialist.

Is it O.K. to exercise alone if you take insulin?

It's always better to have a companion for safety's sake, as well as for company. You especially shouldn't do anything potentially hazardous like skiing or swimming alone.

Still, there isn't always somebody around, and a diabetic does always need his exercise. There's no reason why you can't take a walk or jog or ride your bicycle or play a round of golf by yourself. Just be sure you never leave the house without enough carbohydrate to see you through. *Enough* is the word here. Take along a lot more than you think you can possibly need. Then you'll never have to curtail your fun.

How can I know exactly how much carbohydrate to eat to keep me going through a game of tennis?

If you play right after a meal, eat extra protein at the meal. Protein feeds sugar into the blood slowly for several hours. And, of course, just eat a larger meal.

If you aren't starting your game for as long as two hours after your meal, have a sandwich or a glass of milk or some fruit and cheese. And take along a fast-acting carbohydrate such as fruit juice (pineapple and grape are especially powerful), dried or fresh fruit, candy, sugar, honey, or a soft drink.

You'll have to guess how much of these usually taboo snacks to eat during your game. According to Dr. Joslin, in a tennis match you can take one lump of sugar every twenty minutes.

Other strenuous sports—skiing, basketball, soccer—also require that you start with a big supply of glucose-producers in your stomach, plus a supply in your pocket or knapsack or on the sidelines. Just be sure you take enough and test your urine after two or three ski runs or at the half to make sure you aren't overdoing the carbohydrate.

When the weather is extremely hot or cold, you need more carbohydrate for the same activity. The body's cooling and heating systems require fuel to operate. Ron Santo, third baseman for the Chicago Cubs, told this story on a TV talk show:

> It seemed like a cool day in Chicago. I took a little extra insulin before the game. But it turned out to be a hot day. By the ninth inning, I was getting dizzy. There was a man on first and one on second and I was at bat. I didn't want to cop out, but I was hoping I would strike out, so I could get back to the bench and eat the candy bar the trainer always keeps for me.

Ron didn't strike out. He hit a homer and got back to the dugout in time to eat his candy bar.

Is it all right to drive a car alone on long trips?

Of course. You can do anything anyone else can do. You must, however, always carefully compensate for the behavior of injected insulin. Doctors generally recommend that diabetics at the wheel eat ten grams of carbohydrate every two hours. This means you've got to tote plenty of food along with you in the car.

It should go without saying that when mealtime strikes, stop and dine. If you know there's a dearth of restaurants on the route or if you're particular about what you eat, it's better to take along a picnic meal than to risk having to delay your meal or stoke up on snacks.

How can I keep my insulin the right temperature when I travel?

We've probably been asked this question more often than any other. And the truth of our answer has been doubted more often than that of any other answer we've ever given. Insulin-users simply won't believe that insulin temperature is not all that critical.

The first year June was on insulin she cared for her insulin as if it were a new-born premature infant. On plane flights she would give it to the stewardess to put in the refrigerator and then fret the whole trip for fear she'd forget it. In hotels she was the victim of what we call the old insulin game. She would tip the bellman to put her insulin in the hotel refrigerator and tip him again to fetch it for her, over and over and over again. In ski resorts she'd move her insulin back and forth from dresser to outside on the window ledge so often it was almost as if it were a puppy she was trying to housebreak.

When June finally discussed her complex insulin-temperature-keeping procedures with her doctor, he laughed at her precautions. He particularly laughed at all the insulin ransom money she'd been paying to bellmen. He pointed out that he always carries a bottle of insulin in his medical bag and his bag is left in his car and his car spends most of its time in the San Fernando Valley, an area not known for its summer cool. He said the most that can happen to insulin is that its effectiveness may be slightly diminished.

Of course, if you're planning a three-week summer camping trip in the desert, then it might be a good idea to invest in one of those insulated insulin carriers that sell at exorbitant prices in drugstores or a small wide-mouthed thermos bottle. Otherwise, don't sweat it.

One way, however, that you can really louse up insulin is to freeze it. That's why you shouldn't let it fly with your luggage on planes. The luggage space is sometimes not insulated or pressurized and insulin can freeze there.

Incidentally, you can usually tell if something has gone wrong with insulin by its appearance. If it looks granular or clotted, throw it away. Although its effectiveness may still be as good as ever, it's very difficult to measure and extract the proper dosage when it's in this condition.

Naturally, if you keep an extra bottle of insulin at home, you should keep it in the refrigerator. But you can keep the one you're working with on your dresser or wherever you like without worrying.

As a general rule, just remember the comparison a knowl-

edgeable nurse once made at a diabetes association meeting.
"Your insulin is like your hand. You wouldn't boil your hand
and you wouldn't freeze it. Otherwise, it can take just about
any temperature you can take."

**What do I do about taking insulin when I'm traveling and change time
zones?**

This gives you a great opportunity to prove how flexible
and devious you are. To adjust to a new time zone, you must
either push back your injection time and have an overlap of
insulin coverage, or you must push injection time forward
and have a period of no insulin coverage. The decision is
usually based on whether you leave the United States in the
evening or in the morning and whether you travel east or
west. If you get the feeling that you're stupid when you try
to follow the examples we're going to give you, you're not.
They would confuse an Einstein.

Let's start with a New Yorker flying to Europe, and let's
put him on a 6:00 P.M. dinner flight. Flying time is seven
hours and the time difference between New York and Europe
is six hours. When our New Yorker arrives in Europe, his
watch says 1:00 A.M. but the European clocks all say
7:00 A.M. By the time he gets settled in his hotel (if he was
smart he booked a room for the previous night so that he
could be admitted immediately) it's about 9:00 A.M. European time, but still only 3:00 A.M. New York time. He takes
his injection, even though he's taking it several hours earlier
than his usual schedule.

He may need to take a little less insulin because of the
overlap or eat a little more breakfast. But our New Yorker is
already reestablished on a normal cycle with meal hours
coinciding with his insulin peaks. (Now, his only problem is
trying to stay awake.)

Westerners have a little more to cope with, since the flight
to Europe takes them at least ten and one-half hours, and the
time difference is nine hours. If a Westerner departs on a

morning flight he'll arrive on the morning of the next day, only earlier. If he departs at night, he'll arrive in the late afternoon or early evening, again a day later. By departing at 9:00 A.M., he arrives in Europe at 4:30 A.M.; by departing at 9:00 P.M., he arrives at 4:30 P.M. The choice, then, is to leave at night and miss an entire day, but with the welcome comfort of going to bed soon after arrival.

We prefer to leave at night and arrive in the late afternoon. June then takes one shot of regular insulin, has a light supper, and goes to bed. Next morning she starts her regular injection and meal cycle. If you're on slow-acting insulin and don't want to take one shot of regular to cover supper, you would skip supper, go to bed, and start your usual cycle the next morning.

A Westerner who chooses to leave in the morning and arrive in Europe in the morning can take his injection a few hours after arrival and be back on schedule immediately. In this case he would have an insulin overlap and would need to take less insulin or eat more.

There you have the gist of it. For shorter or longer time differentials, you just juggle in a similar manner. On two- or three-hour time lags you can simply ignore the whole thing. On long sixteen-, eighteen-, and twenty-hour lags, you'll have a chance to hone your juggling skills. Be sure to discuss your plan with your doctor, if you're a novice at this sort of thing.

Questions for Friends and Relatives

My husband wants to think and talk about his diabetes all the time. How can I get him off the subject?

It's hard to find a middle-of-the-road diabetic. Diabetics either try to ignore the disease totally or they become almost obsessed by it. Those who fall into the obsessive category are at least better than the ignorers. They'll probably live longer and eventually outgrow their obsession.

As a matter of fact, many diabetics are only obsessed for a while, right after they're diagnosed. It's not surprising that they should be preoccupied when they first confront a disease that demands the constant attention and thought that diabetes does. A lot of a diabetic's talk about his disease, at this time, is just musing out loud as he tries to figure out what to do; whether he needs another slice of bread to make up for that weeding he did before dinner, if those funny feelings indicate low blood sugar or if they're something totally unrelated to diabetes.

One way that might tone a diabetic down a little is to become more informed on diabetes yourself. By showing the diabetic that you know something about diabetes, he may grow to feel that he can let go of his desperate hammerlock on the subject and relax and let you do some of the thinking for him. If the two of you have workable, give-and-take exchanges on new solutions to his diabetic problems, perhaps he'll be able to cut his personal, lonely fretting time in half and start to think and talk about something else.

Your advantage in knowing something about diabetes is that when he does talk about it, you'll understand what he's saying. Then the talking will seem a lot less like a foreign language you don't understand and, consequently, it will be a lot less boring to you.

If this plan doesn't work or just seems to feed his obsession, then you may eventually have to get tough with him. Tell him in no uncertain terms that nobody loves a monomaniac and that he's going to alienate everybody if he can't talk or think about anything but his disease. This won't be easy to do, especially if you have sympathy and love for the diabetic. Unless somebody sets him straight, however, he's going to ruin his life by thinking of himself as a walking case of diabetes rather than a human being with infinite interests and infinite possibilities who just happens to have diabetes.

How can I tell if a diabetic has low blood sugar?

It helps if you know the diabetic well enough to recognize behavior that isn't normal. If a generally easy-going person starts snapping and snarling, it may be low blood sugar. If a decisive person becomes vague, that can be a clue. Fumbling hands, glassy eyes, slurred speech, perspiration on the forehead or upper lip, a dopey smile, an odd, taut look about the face—all can be symptoms of hypoglycemia (the medical term for low blood sugar). Just about every diabetic has some peculiar signs of his own that you'll grow to recognize, if you're around him a lot and are observant.

Even if you know the person well, though, it's not always easy to recognize low blood sugar. We still remember the time we talked to the Glendale chapter of the Diabetes Association of Southern California about one of our editors who said she could always recognize when June had low blood sugar "because she starts being mean to Barbara." We noticed a woman in the audience frowning. During the question and answer period she said, "My son has diabetes and takes insulin. Often, in fact, very often before dinner he's a holy terror. I can't do a thing with him. Could that be low blood sugar?"

"Oh, boy, could it!" we chorused.

She was really shaken, because she had been punishing him for the misbehavior of his chemicals.

What should I do for a diabetic who has low blood sugar?

First, what you don't do. Don't start a discussion with a diabetic about whether or not he has low blood sugar or what blood-sugar raisers would please his fancy. One of the faculties a diabetic with low blood sugar loses first is his power of decision. While you two sit around chatting about the situation, he grows worse.

A diabetic with low blood sugar also tends to be contentious. He may argue with you both about whether he has low blood sugar or not and what should be eaten to counteract it.

Incidentally, you'd better be pretty well-informed on your diabetic's particular set of low blood sugar symptoms. If you read the clues wrong and load him with carbohydrate when he's grouchy for some reason other than low blood sugar, you'll make him spill. This will blow your credibility with him, and he will never again want to believe you on the subject of low blood sugar, even when he's ready to slip to the floor unconscious from it.

So after you're sure that he has low blood sugar, calmly and forcefully give him something and see that he takes it. (If you're a real friend, you'll *always* carry something in case he forgets.) What should that something be? Well, it should be carbohydrate and it should be fast-acting. If you select something that takes too long to raise the blood sugar, you're likely to keep giving more and more and more, winding up with a gigantic "spill-athon" an hour or so later.

One of our favorite blood sugar raisers is honey. As the headache remedy ads say, it's fast, FAST, *Fast.* It zaps directly into the blood stream. Two teaspoons are the recommended amount. That's just about what you get in one of those handy, little plastic packs of honey that Colonel Sanders packs into his chicken dinner boxes; so you might keep some of those around.

Other good, fast-acting blood sugar raisers are one-half glass of orange juice, one-quarter glass of grape juice, one-half glass of soft drink, two cubes of sugar, one-half candy bar, and two or three Lifesavers or Charms. In camping and hiking stores you can find packs of glucose tablets. These, too, are fast-acting, but they are poorly wrapped and wind up crumbled in the bottom of a purse or pocket. If you buy these tablets, rewrap them individually in foil.

If you become a foxy predictor of low blood sugar attacks and can see them approaching, you can steer your diabetic into a shop which specializes in some delectable blood-sugar raisers—ice cream concoctions, tropical fruit drinks, pastries, etc. On European ski trips, after several runs down the slope, we can clump into the forbidden pastry shop and June can enjoy a strudel or piece of chocolate cake. The pastries in Europe, incidentally, are not nearly so sweet as those in the United States. Often the whipped cream doesn't have a grain of sugar in it. Also, the servings are usually smaller. June's excursions into Alpine pastry shops hardly ever make her spill, even when our low blood sugar estimates are slightly inaccurate.

Warning: Don't keep forcing food down a diabetic until the moment he's back to normal. It takes at least ten or fifteen minutes for the body to react. Have him sit down or lie down until he feels better. Unless there's a meal coming up, give him a snack of slower-acting carbohydrate or a carbohydrate and protein combination after he recuperates.

What should I do if I find a diabetic unconscious?

Unconsciousness can be either diabetic coma, which means the diabetic has too much sugar, or insulin shock, which means he has too little.

If you know the diabetic takes insulin and sticks to his diet pretty well, then you can be almost certain it's insulin shock. If you know how to give an injection and where the diabetic keeps his glucagon, you can give him a shot of that. If you have a tube of instant glucose (available from some drugstores or from the Diabetes Association of Cleveland, 2980 Mayfield Road, Cleveland Heights, Ohio 44118), you can squeeze a little inside his cheek. *Never,* under any circumstances, pour any liquid like fruit juice or Coca Cola down his throat, as it could wind up in his lungs and suffocate him. If you can't do either of these things, then you can give him a sugar solution enema. With any of these methods the diabetic should come around in about fifteen minutes. In cases where none of the above treatments is available to you, call a doctor.

If you know for sure that the diabetic doesn't take insulin or pills and doesn't follow his diet or take care of himself, then he's probably in diabetic coma, the long-range result of diabetic misbehavior. In this case, call his doctor or an ambulance immediately. There's nothing much you can do for him. He needs massive insulin doses of the kind that can only be given in a hospital.

If you have no idea whether you're dealing with insulin shock or diabetic coma, treat for insulin shock. If it's diabetic coma, the diabetic already has so much sugar floating through his system that a little more isn't going to make all that much difference. And if it *is* insulin shock, your quick treatment could be a lifesaver. A person in good health will eventually come out of insulin shock on his own, but for someone with a heart condition the shock could prove disastrous.

If my diabetic child goes to a birthday party or trick or treating on Halloween, is it all right for him to break his diet just this once?

No. Think how many "just this once's" that would make in a year. Before long, just this once becomes an everyday occurrence and horrible habits are established. Your child's health and maybe even his life expectancy are diminished.

It's hard to see your child deprived, when other kids are loading up on goodies—maybe it's even harder on you than on him—but diabetes is going to be with him all his life. Now is when the lifetime behavior patterns are established. You're *not* being kind when you let him break his diet just this once.

We still recall with fear and trembling the story of one "kind" father, who also fancied himself such an expert in diabetes that he could smash all the rules to smithereens. We heard his story when he was appearing on a diabetes panel, and we sat there marveling that no one rose up in wrath to stuff his mouth with cotton balls and Tes-Tape. This person didn't want his little girl to miss out on the carbohydratous joys of Halloween. He instructed her, before she went out, to please remember everything she ate on her trick-or-treat rounds. When she got home, he gave her a wallop of regular insulin to cover it all. He seemed to believe he could calculate exactly the right amount of insulin to compensate for the candy. He actually spoke of what he did with pride and recommended it as an ideal solution. This struck us as being similar to saying proudly that you'd been slipping a little arsenic in your child's cereal.

One thing you can do on occasions when your child is being deprived is figure out some way he can get extra attention. Attention is an even more satisfying commodity to the young (or the middle-aged and old, for that matter) than ice cream and cake and candy. Let him pass out the forbidden food to others in much the same way that some alcoholics like to act as bartender at parties. On Halloween let him organize a door-to-door collection for UNICEF. Use your imagination to help him stay on his diet, instead of your pity to help him break it just this once.

Should I give up eating pastries so my diabetic husband won't feel tempted?

Admittedly, it's a little hard to sit there and wolf down a huge slab of banana cream pie, if your husband is watching you like a spaniel. You both feel sorry for him, you feel guilty, and these are very digestion-upsetting emotions. Still, you definitely shouldn't give up your pastries for your husband's sake. He's going to have to get used to being tempted and resisting temptation. It's similar to an alcoholic's situation. He has to be able to go to a place where others are drinking and yet not drink himself.

There remains, however, a question you didn't ask. And that is, should you give up pastries for your *own* sake? Pastries are hardly the nutritional dream dish for anybody, diabetic or not. And how is *your* weight?

My father has diabetes. Is there any way I can keep from getting it?

Act as if you already have it. Follow the diabetic regime. Stay away from concentrated sweets. Eat the diabetic diet. Keep your weight slightly below normal. Get plenty of exercise. (It's always easier to follow a regime like the diabetic one, if you don't have to.)

Even if you aren't programmed to get diabetes, you'll feel terrific and probably will increase your life span because of your healthy regime. If diabetes is in the cards for you (if one of your parents has diabetes, you have a 22 percent chance of getting it), you may be able to prevent or at least delay its appearance. If you do develop diabetes, you'll already know how to handle it and will have established good diabetic habits. Adjusting to the disease will be no problem at all for you.

How can I help my child accept his diabetes?

First, accept it yourself. Children are great little chameleons. They pick up the attitudes and emotions of parents faster than you can say Banting and Best. If you have the attitude that your child's diabetes is a disaster and a loathsome burden, that's the attitude your child will develop. If you take his diabetes in your stride, accept the restrictions of the disease, and work positively toward helping him learn how to lead that proverbial normal life, you'll instill these positive attitudes in him by living example.

Incidentally, your question hit on the number one, foremost, important adjustment attitude for a diabetic— acceptance. It may be the hardest to come by, but once acceptance is there, all the rest is relatively easy.

Should I give my husband his insulin injections?

Yes and no. Yes, you should give them to him sometimes. You can reach injection sites he can't reach himself, unless he's a contortionist. This is a big help. Since a diabetic isn't suppose to inject within one inch of the same spot for a month, you can see how easily he can run out of accessible areas, especially if he has to shoot more than once a day.

Another reason for giving him his insulin is that you'll know how to give an injection. Should he ever pass out in insulin shock, you'll know how to give him glucagon, which is injected in the same way as insulin, and bring him out of it.

But no, you shouldn't *always* give him his injection. He's got to be mainly responsible for his own insulin shooting. No one should be that dependent on another person. It's almost like being dependent on another person for your breathing. It's not good for him nor for you, either.

We know a nurse whose husband is a diabetic. At first, he tried to wheedle her into giving him his shot every day. He got nowhere with her. She was as firm as Senator Inouye's nurse after he had had his arm amputated in Italy during the war. The senator's nurse handed him a pack of cigarettes and matches but refused to either open the pack or light the match. She explained, "I'm not always going to be around to do things for you. You're going to have to learn to do for yourself."

If I mention my wife's diabetes in a restaurant to try to get her something special, like a substitute for sweet and sour pork in a Chinese dinner, she gets furious and says I make her feel like a freak. What can I do?

This answer is simplicity itself. You say to the waiter, "I am a diabetic and I can't eat anything with sugar in it. Could we please substitute pork with Chinese greens for the sweet and sour pork?" By claiming to be the diabetic yourself, you take the burden of asking for special favors off your wife's conscience, or pride, or whatever area of her psychological being is disturbed.

After you've claimed to be the diabetic for a while, maybe your wife will wise up to the fact 'that having diabetes is nothing to be ashamed of. She'll come to realize that, for the most part, people in restaurants as well as in other walks of life are usually happy to help out with little problems associated with diabetes. This is an important step in her acceptance of her disease.

What should I do if we're out dining in a restaurant and my husband, who is diabetic, orders all the wrong things for himself?

Diabetics sometimes perversely do this. Even June, who is the most careful and rational of diabetics, has occasionally suffered this restaurant aberration.

The best thing to do when you hear the diabetically inappropriate meal being ordered is not to screech and rant and embarrass your husband in front of the waiter, but rather to order a diabetic back-up meal for yourself. Usually when his meal is presented to him, the diabetic takes one look at it and comes to his senses. Then you just say casually, without any lectures or recriminations, "It looks as if my dinner might be better for you than yours. Would you like to trade?" The diabetic almost always will with gratitude. (Probably as much gratitude for the freedom from lectures and recriminations as for the food.)

Naturally, to perform this little sleight of plate act, you have to know what a diabetically appropriate meal is. But if you cook for your husband, you probably know as well or better than he does.

My son wants to play football. Is that safe for a diabetic?

There have been several outstanding diabetic football players. Ron Mix of the University of Southern California and Coley O'Brien of Notre Dame are just two. No diabetic evil ever befell them because of football. If your son's diabetes is without complications and in good control, then there is no earthly reason why he shouldn't play.

There are two good reasons why he should. Participation in sports, especially a physically demanding one like football, will encourage him to take superb care of himself and his disease. For a young person, the incentive to keep in shape for football is far more powerful than a general incentive to watch one's health. Once your son has established good habits during his football-playing days, there's a fair chance he'll stick with them throughout his life.

He should be allowed to play football for psychological reasons as well. If his diabetes keeps him from playing football, he'll get the idea that because of diabetes he can't do anything. On the other hand, if he plays football, his attitude will more likely be that, despite his diabetes, he can do everything he really wants to. Which attitude would you prefer him to carry through life?

Be sure that he informs the coach and his teammates that he has diabetes and explains to them what they should do in case he has an insulin reaction.

And, finally, do your best not to show excessive concern every time he goes out to play, even if you feel it way down inside your own pancreas. If you load him up with your fears and negative vibes, you'll wreck his game and maybe cause an accident rather than prevent one. A football player needs a positive attitude above all else and so does a diabetic.

Should I hire a diabetic?

We'll answer that question with another question. Is the diabetic the most qualified person you're considering for the job? If your answer is yes, then our answer to you is yes.

Eighty-five percent of all diabetics, those not taking insulin, can handle any job that any other person can and do it just as safely and well.

The 15 percent who do take insulin should not work at anything in which they might threaten the safety of others or themselves, should they have an insulin reaction on the job. This would include jobs such as flying or operating dangerous machinery. But probably no insulin-taking diabetic would apply for such a job. All other work areas are, or should be, open to them.

One advantage in hiring a diabetic is that he'll never have to take the day off with a hangover.

How do I plan a meal for my diabetic friend?

Just remember that a diabetic has to stay away from concentrated sweets—sugar, honey, molasses in or on foods, and canned fruit in sweet syrup. Remember also that starches—crackers, bread, potatoes, corn, rice, flour—contain carbohydrates, which a diabetic can eat only in limited quantities. Go easy on them. This doesn't mean you have to eliminate them entirely. A diabetic, especially one who takes insulin, has to have a specific amount of carbohydrate in his diet. Just have something like bread, rice, or potatoes available, and the diabetic will know how much he can have.

That's another point to remember. Just as important as what is allowed is how much. A diabetic must limit the quantities of food he eats. Don't be offended if your diabetic friend eats with gusto and then suddenly stops, as if someone has blown a whistle on him. He hasn't found a bug in his food. It's just that he's eaten all he is allowed. Don't urge him to eat more. That's being cruel. He'd probably love to eat more, and it's taking all his will power to stop.

A basic diabetic meal would be something like this: a mixed green salad; meat or chicken or fish; potatoes or bread or rice; a vegetable or two (*not* corn and *not* any kind of beans except green beans); and fruit for dessert (either fresh or canned without sugar). Now, on the surface this may sound pretty blah, but any and all of these elements can be combined in something like beef stroganoff or bouillabaisse or chicken marengo or lamb curry. Just remember, generally, what ingredients you put into the dish and tell the diabetic so he can estimate his portions.

Technically, a diabetic is supposed to have milk with his meal, but many prefer to use it as a between-meal snack or don't care for it; instead, they have cheese and fruit, which amounts to the same thing as milk in the diet. Ask your friend what he prefers. If he's not a milk-drinker, one thing you can do is use the cheese in a dip for an appetizer. If you use a cheese dip, you might serve it with carrot or celery sticks or thin slices of turnip for dipping, rather than the usual carbohydrate-laden potato or corn chips and crackers.

If your diabetic friend drinks, be sure you don't offer him only sweet mixers (ginger ale, 7-Up, tonic) or serve him some kind of fruit punch. The fruit juice adds carbohydrates almost as fast as pure sugar. A diabetic can drink noncarbohydrous liquors such as gin, vodka, scotch, bourbon, dry vermouth, and dry sherry. He can have these either straight or with water, plain soda, or artificially sweetened mixers. Don't give a diabetic more than a standard jigger with the idea that you're being generous. In fact, the best thing you can do is let him fix his own drink, so he'll know exactly how much he's getting. And don't urge more alcohol on a diabetic any more than you'd urge more food on him.

Actually, drinking alcohol is highly controversial for a diabetic. Some doctors forbid it totally, and even the doctors who permit drinking permit only very small quantities.

If you plan to have wine with dinner, make sure it's dry wine. Sweet wines have carbohydrates. Tell your diabetic friend that you're having wine so he can decide to skip anything alcoholic before dinner or have a half measure in order to have a little wine with the meal. And don't offer a diabetic a sweet liqueur after dinner; they're verboten because of the sugar in them.

As you can see, the most important thing is to let the

diabetic know what's going on. Surprises are fun, but not for a diabetic who's trying to plot his diet. Take him aside and give him a preview of the meal or give it to him on the telephone beforehand. This will allow him to relax and enjoy himself.

If your diabetic friend is on insulin (ask!), then you should tell him what time you're serving. This doesn't mean what time the guests are arriving, but what time you'll actually have everybody sitting at the table with food on their plates. Then, once you've told him the time, *stick to that time,* no matter who hasn't arrived by then (except, of course, the diabetic himself). Once a diabetic on insulin takes his morning shot, he's locked into a rigid schedule of eating times and he can get in trouble, maybe even go into insulin shock, if he doesn't eat meals when he should. His only alternative, if you stall the meal on him, is to fill up on any snacks you have around, and then he'll have used up most of his dinner quota of food and will only be able to pick at the meal. This is an unhealthy eating pattern for him and a disturbing experience for both of you.

One thing you shouldn't do is restrict other guests to the diabetic diet. It doesn't make a diabetic happy to feel that others are being deprived on his account. He sees plenty of diabetically forbidden food go down other people's hatches all the time. He's used to it. If you normally serve both bread and potatoes or rice or some kind of pasta dish, go right ahead. The diabetic can select which he prefers, or maybe he'll have a half serving of each. If you normally serve some kind of wild, sweet dessert, go ahead with that, too. Just have a piece of fruit for the diabetic.

We've rambled on this topic, probably making it sound more complicated than it really is. A diabetic meal is, in actuality, not all that different from a nondiabetic one. (For general dietetic information, see Appendix M.) If you're still confused about anything on the diabetic diet, just follow the advice of all the sex manual writers who say, "If in doubt about what will please your partner, *ask!"*

My little boy has had temper tantrums since his diabetes was diagnosed. Is this normal?

No. If his temper tantrums occur at the same time every day, especially if that time is always just before meals, it could be insulin reaction. If, however, his tantrums come at all times, the cause may not be his diabetes so much as your reaction to his diabetes. Because of pity or fear or guilt or a combination of the three, you may be pampering and indulging him into perfect "bratdom."

It's understandable that you're disturbed over having, in some way, transmitted diabetes to your child and that you want to make it up to him. But think how much worse you'll feel if you discover in later years that, with the very best of intentions, you have turned him into a rotten human being.

The damage you do may not be just to him, either. All the other members of your family may well build up resentments over always having to play second fiddle to the diabetic virtuoso.

Naturally, you should first report the problem to your doctor and make sure there isn't some physical reason for your son's tantrums. If there isn't, *you* may be the one with the behavior problem.

My daughter is diabetic. How can I find out more about diabetes and how to help her?

You can read the first part of this book and other books you can find on the subject. You can attend one of the diabetes education programs in your community (see page 13). You can subscribe to publications on diabetes (see page 19). And if there is a diabetes association in your community, you can join it and attend all the meetings.

Then, as soon as your daughter is old enough to start assimilating information, you can begin feeding it to her and encouraging her to learn more on her own. It's admirable to help her, but even more admirable to help her help herself.

For a starter you can write for a copy of *Mr. Hypo Is My Friend,* a free educational booklet for young children, distributed by the Ames Company (Division Miles Laboratories, Inc., Elkhart, Indiana 46514). Eli Lilly and Company (Indianapolis, Indiana 46206), publishes a comic book, *Keith and Tommy Climb to a New Life,* for slightly older children. If there is a diabetes summer camp for children in your area (ask the local diabetes association), that is one of the best ways for children to learn more about diabetes and have fun doing it.

When my husband has low blood sugar, he gets very hostile and disagreeable. How can I keep from reacting to him and getting angry myself?

If you're a normal human being, you probably can't always. In the first place, you can't always know for sure that he's acting disagreeable because of low blood sugar, unless, of course, he's some kind of a saint who never, never says an unkind word to you. And in the second place, you may flare up at him before it even crosses your mind that it's his chemistry that's attacking you.

Barbara has known June every minute of the seven years she'e had diabetes and she's known her for another seven years before that. She's as familiar as anyone could be with June's normal personality. And yet, when June starts being rude and insulting and belligerent, Barbara's hackles rise and she gets mad right back, until it suddenly dawns on her that June is not acting normal and needs, not the split lip she feels like giving her, but some fast-acting carbohydrate.

Just recently the head librarian where we work was consulting us on our work schedules for the next semester. June snarled, "We can't possibly give you an answer. Barbara wants to change the schedule every other week. You can't pin her down on anything." Barbara reared back and hotly defended herself against the accusation. And then pausing in mid-rant, she said, "I think you have low blood sugar." June replied, "I probably do." Off went Barbara and the head librarian for a couple of fast-acting fig bars.

After June had chomped them down, Barbara immediately said, *"Now,* let's decide about our schedule." But June still couldn't get her wits together to analyze the possibilities. Barbara had made the classic mistake: it takes fifteen or so minutes, depending on exactly how low the blood sugar is, for a diabetic to regain his rationality. Barbara knows this full well, but unfortunately we don't always act on our knowledge. Nobody does, diabetic or nondiabetic, but we can all keep trying.

Appendix

Appendix A

Affiliate Association of the
American Diabetes Association

American Diabetes Association, Inc.
18 East 48th Street
New York, New York 10017

Alabama   Alabama Diabetes Association, Inc.
           3005 North Woodridge
           Birmingham, Alabama 35203

Alaska   Alaska Diabetes Association, Inc.
           P.O. Box 4495
           Anchorage, Alaska 99503

California Northern California Diabetes Association, Inc.
            255 Hugo Street
            San Francisco, California 94122
            Telephone: 415 681-0210

            Diabetes Association of Southern California, Inc.
            4849 Van Nuys Boulevard
            Sherman Oaks, California 91403
            Telephone: 213 872-1385 or 986-6272

Colorado   Colorado Diabetes Association, Inc.
           1375 Delaware Street
           Denver, Colorado 80204
           Telephone: 303 573-7000

Connecticut

Connecticut Diabetes Association, Inc.
47 College Street - Room 230
New Haven, Connecticut 06510
Telephone: 203 776-4685

Delaware

Delaware Diabetes Association, Inc.
1925 Lovering Avenue
Wilmington, Delaware 19806
Telephone: 302 656-0030

District of
Columbia

Diabetes Association of the Washington D.C.
Metropolitan Area, Inc.
P.O. Box 4384, Takoma Park Branch
Washington, D.C. 20012
Telephone: 301 681-5930

Florida

Florida Diabetes Association, Inc.
P.O. Box 2003
Jacksonville, Florida 30203

Georgia

Georgia Diabetes Association, Inc.
762 Cypress Street, N.E.
Atlanta, Georgia 30308
Telephone: 404 874-5875

Illinois

Diabetes Association of Greater Chicago, Inc.
620 North Michigan Avenue
Chicago, Illinois 60611
Telephone: 312 943-8668

Downstate Illinois Diabetes Association, Inc.
100 West Miller Street
Springfield, Illinois 62702
Telephone: 217 544-9881
Thomas D. Masters, M.D., President

Idaho

Idaho Diabetes Association, Inc.
2400 Bella Street
Boise, Idaho 83702

Indiana	Indiana Diabetes Association, Inc. 810 Hume Mansur Building Indianapolis, Indiana 46204 Telephone: 317 639-1111
Kansas	Contact Missouri State Diabetes Association, Inc.
Kentucky	Kentucky Diabetes Association, Inc. Department of Pediatrics Room MN-480 University of Kentucky Medical Center Lexington, Kentucky 40506
Louisiana	Diabetes Association of Louisiana, Inc. 1121 Louisiana Avenue Shreveport, Louisiana 71101 Telephone: 318 422-2158
Maine	See Massachusetts
Maryland	Maryland Diabetes Association, Inc. 407 Reisterstown Road Pikesville, Maryland 21208 Telephone: 301 358-2445
Massachusetts	New England Diabetes Association, Inc. 1223 Beacon St., Room 107 Brookline, Massachusetts 02146 Telephone: 617 731-2972
Michigan	Michigan Diabetes Association, Inc. 6131 West Outer Drive Detroit, Michigan 48235 Telephone: 313 342-9333
Minnesota	Twin Cities Diabetes Association, Inc. W-116 Meadowbrook Medical Building 6490 Excelsior Boulevard Minneapolis, Minnesota 55426 Telephone: 612 927-4487

Mississippi	Diabetes Association of Mississippi, Inc. 1126 Adkins Boulevard Jackson, Mississippi 39211
Missouri	Missouri State Diabetes Association, Inc. 303 Spring Fayette, Missouri 65248
Montana	Montana Diabetes Association, Inc. P.O. Box 2088 Great Falls, Montana 59401
Nebraska	Nebraska Diabetes Association, Inc. c/o Department of Medicine University of Nebraska College of Medicine 42nd and Dewey Omaha, Nebraska 68105
Nevada	Nevada Diabetes Association, Inc. 17 Ben Rea Circle Las Vegas, Nevada 89110
New Hampshire	See Massachusetts
New Jersey	New Jersey Diabetes Association, Inc. 317 Belleville Avenue Bloomfield, New Jersey 07003 Telephone: 201 748-6490
New Mexico	New Mexico Diabetes Association, Inc. 1441 Wyoming Boulevard Albuquerque, New Mexico 87112
New York	Buffalo Diabetes Association, Inc. Kenmore Mercy Hospital 2950 Elmwood Avenue Buffalo, New York 14217

New York Diabetes Association, Inc.
104 East 40th Street
New York, New York 10016
Telephone: 212 OXford 7-7760

Niagara Falls Diabetes Association, Inc.
457 3rd Street
Niagara Falls, New York 14301

Rochester Regional Diabetes Association, Inc.
1351 Mount Hope Avenue
Rochester, New York 14620
Telephone: 716 271-4220

North Carolina North Carolina Diabetes Association, Inc.
408 North Tryon Street
Charlotte, North Carolina 28202
Telephone: 704 333-1568

North Dakota North Dakota Diabetes Association, Inc.
221 South Fourth Street
Grand Forks, North Dakota 58201
Telephone: 701 775-8121

Ohio Diabetes Association of the Cincinnati Area, Inc.
2400 Reading Road
Cincinnati, Ohio 45202
Telephone: 513 721-3160

Dayton Area Diabetes Association, Inc.
184 Salem Avenue
Dayton, Ohio 45406
Telephone: 513 461-5810

Greater Akron Area Diabetes Association, Inc.
326 Locust Street
Akron, Ohio 44302
Telephone: 216 253-1171

Oklahoma	Oklahoma Diabetes Association, Inc. 2021 South Lewis Tulsa, Oklahoma 74104 Telephone: 918 742-3361
Pennsylvania	Delaware Valley Diabetes Association, Inc. 332 South 13th Street - 3rd Floor Philadelphia, Pennsylvania 19107 Telephone: 215 PEnnypacker 5-2541
	Lehigh Valley Diabetes Association, Inc. 1434 North Broad Street Allentown, Pennsylvania 18104
	Pittsburgh Diabetes Association, Inc. 200 Ross Street Pittsburgh, Pennsylvania 15219 Telephone: 412 261-6010, Extension 306
	Reading Diabetes Association, Inc. 2305 Gring Drive - Whitfield Reading, Pennsylvania 19609
Rhode Island	See Massachusetts
South Carolina	South Carolina Diabetes Association, Inc. c/o Medical College of South Carolina 80 Barre Street Charleston, South Carolina 29401
Tennessee	Tennessee Diabetes Association, Inc. c/o Diabetes Education Program 530 Medical Arts Building Nashville, Tennessee 37212 Telephone: 615 322-3357
Texas	Dallas Diabetes Association, Inc. 4232 Herschel Street Dallas, Texas 75219 Telephone: 214 RIverside 7-2185

South Texas Diabetes Association, Inc.
P.O. Box 1638
Pasadena, Texas 77501
Telephone 713 941-8437

Vermont   See Massachusetts

Virginia   Virginia Diabetes Association, Inc.
University of Virginia Hospital
Box 145
Charlottesville, Virginia 22901

Washington   Washington Diabetes Association, Inc.
1000 Seneca Street
Seattle, Washington 98101
Telephone: 206 MAin 4-5240

West Virginia   West Virginia Diabetes Association, Inc.
1033 Forest Road
Charleston, West Virginia 25314
Telephone: 304 343-2743

Wisconsin   Wisconsin Diabetes Association, Inc.
225 East Michigan Street
Milwaukee, Wisconsin 53202
Telephone: 414 276-6447

Appendix B

Recommended Weight for Diabetics

HEIGHT-WEIGHT TABLES
FOR YOUNG MEN AND WOMEN

Overweight has been defined as 15 to 30 per cent above average weight, obesity as more than 30 per cent above average weight. Until recently it has been more difficult to define one extreme opposite. Analyses of height-weight come from about 150,000 college students provide tables which include figures for the underweight. Study of the students indicated that weight was relatively stable between 21 and 29 years for men and between ages 17 and 29 for women.

YOUNG MEN

Height (in.)	Under-weight	Slender	Normal	Stocky	Over-weight	Obese
63	111	121	131	141	151	170
64	114	124	134	144	155	175
65	117	128	138	148	159	179
66	120	131	141	152	163	184
67	123	134	145	156	167	188
68	126	138	149	160	171	193
69	130	141	152	164	175	198
70	133	145	156	168	180	203
71	136	148	160	172	184	209
72	140	152	165	177	189	214
73	143	156	169	181	194	219
74	147	160	173	186	199	225
75	151	164	178	191	204	231
76	155	168	182	196	209	237
77	159	173	187	201	215	243
78	163	177	192	206	220	249

YOUNG WOMEN

Height (in.)	Under- weight	Slender	Normal	Stocky	Over- weight	Obese
58	88	95	103	111	119	134
59	90	98	106	114	122	138
60	93	101	109	117	125	142
61	95	104	112	120	129	146
62	98	106	115	124	132	150
63	101	109	118	127	136	154
64	103	112	122	131	140	158
65	106	116	125	134	144	162
66	109	119	128	138	148	167
67	112	122	132	142	152	172
68	115	126	136	146	156	176
69	119	129	140	150	160	181
70	122	133	143	154	165	186
71	125	136	147	158	170	192
72	129	140	152	163	174	197
73	132	144	156	167	179	202
74	136	148	160	172	184	208

*Underweight = 15 per cent or less of average weight

Slender = 7.5 to -15 per cent of average weight

Normal = average weight computed for men from the equation, $W = 26.7_e^{0.0253H}$ and for women, $W = 9.50_e^{0.0108H}$

Stocky = +7.5 to +15 per cent of average weight

Overweight = +15 per cent to +30 per cent of average weight

Obese = +30 per cent or more of average weight

(Dorothy W. Sargent, M.S.: "Weight-height relationship of young men and women," *American Journal of Clinical Nutrition*, November 1963.)

Appendix C
Food Exchange Lists

General Rules

Eat your meals about the same time every day. Eat only the amounts given on your diet plan and do not skip meals.

Measuring food: Food should be measured. You will need a standard 8-ounce measuring cup and a measuring teaspoon and tablespoon. All measurements are level. Cooked foods are measured after being cooked.

Food preparation: Meats should be baked, boiled, roasted or broiled (indoors or on an outdoor grill). Do not fry foods unless fat allowed in meal is used.

Fat allowed on your diet may be used to season vegetables. Vegetables may be cooked in bouillon or fat-free meat broth if desired.

Food selection: Select your diet from the same foods purchased for the rest of the family—milk, vegetables, bread, meats, fats, and fruit (fresh, dried, or frozen or canned without sugar).

Many special dietetic foods should not be used unless they are figured in the diet plan. Always check the labels of these foods for protein, carbohydrate, fat, and calorie content.

Foods to be avoided unless permitted by your doctor:

sugar	pie
candy	cake
honey	cookies
jam	pastries
jelly	condensed milk
marmalade	soft drinks (regular)
syrups	candy-coated gum

fried, scalloped, or creamed foods
beer, wine, or other alcoholic beverages

Use of the exchange lists is based on the recommendations of the American Diabetes Association and the American Dietetic Association in cooperation with the Diabetes Branch of the U.S. Public Health Service, Department of Health, Education, and Welfare.

Food Exchange Lists

List 1: Allow as Desired
(need not be measured)

Seasonings: Celery salt, cinnamon, garlic, garlic salt, lemon, mint, mustard, nutmeg, parsley, pepper, saccharin and other noncaloric sweeteners, spices, vanilla, and vinegar.

Other foods: Coffee or tea (without sugar or cream), diet beverage without sugar, fat-free broth, bouillon, unflavored gelatin, artificially sweetened fruit-flavored gelatin, sour or dill pickles, cranberries or rhubarb (without sugar).

Vegetables: Group A—insignificant carbohydrates or calories. You may eat as much raw vegetable as desired. Limit total amount of cooked vegetable or vegetables to 1 cup.

asparagus	lettuce
broccoli	mushrooms
brussels sprouts	okra
cabbage	peppers, green or red

cauliflower
celery
chicory
cucumbers
eggplant
escarole
greens: beet, chard,
    collard, dandelion, kale,
    mustard, spinach, turnip

radishes
sauerkraut
squash, summer
string beans
tomatoes
watercress

List 2: Vegetable Exchanges

Each portion supplies approximately 7 grams of carbohydrate and 2 grams of protein, or 36 calories.

Vegetables: Group B—one serving equals 1/2 cup, or 100 grams.

beets
carrots
onions

peas, green
pumpkin
rutabagas

squash, winter
turnips

List 3: Fruit Exchanges

(fresh, dried, or frozen or canned without sugar or syrup)

Each portion supplies approximately 10 grams of carbohydrate, or 40 calories.

	Measurement
apple	1 small (2″ diam.)
apple juice	1/3 cup
applesauce	1/2 cup
apricots, fresh	2 med.
apricots, dried	4 halves
banana	1/2 small
berries (boysenberries, blackberries, raspberries, strawberries)	1 cup

blueberries	2/3 cup
cantaloupe	1/4 (6″ diam.)
cherries	10 large
dates	2
figs, fresh	2 large
figs, dried	1 small
fruit cocktail	1/2 cup
grapefruit	1/2 small
grapefruit juice	1/2 cup
grapes	12
grape juice	1/4 cup
honeydew melon	1/8 (7″)
mandarin oranges	3/4 cup
mango	1/2 small
nectarine	1 small
orange	1 small
orange juice	1/2 cup
papaya	1/3 med.
peach	1 med.
pear	1 small
pineapple	1/2 cup
pineapple juice	1/3 cup
plums	2 med.
prunes, dried	2
prune juice	1/4 cup
raisins	2 tbsp.
tangerine	1 large
watermelon	1 cup

List 4: Bread Exchanges

Each portion supplies approximately 15 grams of carbohydrate and 2 grams of protein, or 68 calories.

	Measurement
bread	1 slice
bagel	1/2
biscuit, roll	1 (2" diam.)
bun (for hamburger or wiener) . .	1/2
cornbread	1-1/2" cube
English muffin	1/2
muffin	1 (2" diam.)
cake, angel or sponge, without icing	1-1/2" cube (1/20 of 10"-diam. cake)
cereal, cooked	1/2 cup
dry (flakes or puffed)	3/4 cup
cornstarch	2 tbsp.
crackers, graham	2 (2-1/2" sq.)
oyster	20 (1/2 cup)
round	6
saltine	5
variety	5 small
flour	2-1/2 tbsp.
matzo	1 (6" diam.)
popcorn, popped, unbuttered	1 cup
rice or grits, cooked	1/2 cup
spaghetti, macaroni, noodles, cooked	1/2 cup
vegetables	
beans, baked, without pork . . .	1/4 cup
lima, navy, etc., dry, cooked . .	1/2 cup
corn	1/3 cup
corn on the cob	1/2 med. ear
parsnips	2/3 cup
peas (split peas, etc.), dry, cooked	1/2 cup
potatoes, sweet, or yams, fresh . .	1/4 cup
white, baked or boiled	1 (2" diam.)
white, mashed	1/2 cup

List 5: Meat Exchanges

Each portion supplies approximately 7 grams of protein and 5 grams of fat, or 73 calories.

	Measurement
Cheese, cheddar, American	1-oz. slice (3-1/2" sq., 1/8" thick)
cottage	1/4 cup
egg	1
fish and seafood	
halibut, perch, sole, etc.	1-oz. slice (4" x 2" x 1/4")
oysters, clams, shrimp	5 small
salmon, tuna, crab	1/4 cup
sardines	3 med.
meat and poultry	
beef, lamb, pork, veal, ham, liver, chicken, etc. (med. fat)	1-oz. slice (4" x 2" x 1/4")
cold cuts	1-1/2 oz. slice (4-1/2" sq., 1/8" thick)
Vienna sausages	2
*wiener	1 (10 per lb.)
*peanut butter	2 tbsp.

*Limit peanut butter and wieners to one exchange per day.

List 6: Fat Exchanges

Each portion supplies approximately 5 grams of fat, or 45 calories.

	Measurement
avocado	1/8 (4″ diam.)
bacon, crisp	1 slice
butter or margarine	1 tsp.
cream, half and half	3 tbsp.
heavy, 40%	1 tbsp.
light, 20%	2 tbsp.
sour	2 tbsp.
cream cheese	1 tbsp.
dressing, French	1 tbsp.
mayonnaise	1 tsp.
roquefort	2 tsp.
nuts	6 small
oil or cooking fat	1 tsp.
olives	5 small

List 7: Milk Values

Each portion supplies approximately 12 grams of carbohydrate and 8 grams of protein; the fat content and total calories vary with the type of milk. (One fat exchange equals 5 grams of fat.)

	Measurement	Fat exchanges	Calories
milk			
buttermilk	1 cup	—	80
evaporated, undiluted	1/2 cup	2	170
nonfat dry milk mixed according to directions on box	1 cup	—	80

nonfat dry milk powder	1/4 cup	—	80
skim	1 cup	—	80
2% butterfat	1 cup	1	125
whole	1 cup	2	170
yogurt, plain, made with skim milk	1 cup	1	125

If you want to make a substitution in the milk called for in your diet plan, either choose a milk product that contains the same number of fat exchanges or allow for the difference in your meal plan. For example, if your diet plan calls for 1 cup of 2% milk (1 fat exchange), you may substitute 1 cup of buttermilk (no fat) plus one additional fat exchange.

Miscellaneous Foods

The following foods may be used in your diet if you wish. They must be figured into the daily diet plan, with the food exchanges allowed as indicated.

	Measurement	Exchanges
chili sauce	1 tbsp.	1 list 2 vegetable
fish sticks, frozen	3 sticks	1 bread, 2 meat
fruit-flavored gelatin	1/4 cup	1 bread
ginger ale	7 oz.	1 bread
ice cream, vanilla, chocolate, strawberry	1/2 cup	1 bread, 2 fat
low-calorie dressing, French of Italian	1 tbsp.	—†
potato chips	10 large or 15 small	1 bread 2 fat
sherbet	1/2 cup	2 bread

vanilla wafers	6	1 bread
waffle, frozen	1 (5-1/2")	1 bread

†The fat and calorie content do not have to be counted if the amount is limited to 1 tablespoonful.

—Courtesy of Eli Lilly and Company

Appendix D
Daily Menu Guides

These sample menus show some of the ways that the exchange lists may be used to add variety to your meals. **Use the exchange lists to plan different menus.**

Daily Menu Guide: 1000 Calories

Breakfast:	**Breakfast Example:**	
1 fruit exchange (list 3)	orange juice	1/2 cup
1 bread exchange (list 4)	toast	1 slice
1 meat exchange (list 5)	egg	1
1/2 cup skim milk (list 7)	skim milk	1/2 cup

Lunch:	**Lunch Example:**	
2 meat exchanges (list 5)	cheese	2 1-oz. slices
1 bread exchange (list 4)	bread	1 slice
vegetable(s) as desired (list 1)	tomato salad	as desired
1 fruit exchange (list 3)	apple	1 small
1/2 cup skim milk (list 7)	skim milk	1/2 cup
1 fat exchange (list 6)	mayonnaise	1 tsp.

Dinner:	**Dinner Example:**	
3 meat exchanges (list 5)	chicken, baked	3 oz.
1/2 bread exchange (list 4)	potatoes, mashed	1/4 cup
vegetable(s) as desired (list 1)	salad from list 1 vegetables	as desired
1 vegetable exchange (list 2)	peas	1/2 cup
1 fruit exchange (list 3)	fruit cocktail	1/2 cup
1 fat exchange (list 6)	margarine	1 tsp.

Bedtime Feeding:	**Bedtime Feeding Example:**	
1 cup skim milk (list 7)	skim milk	1 cup
or	or	
1 fruit exchange (list 3)	grapefruit juice	1/2 cup
1/2 bread exchange (list 4)	graham cracker	1 square

Daily Menu Guide: 1200 Calories

Breakfast:
1 fruit exchange (list 3)
1-1/2 bread exchanges (list 4)

1 meat exchange (list 5)
1/2 cup 2% milk (list 7)
1 fat exchange (list 6)

Breakfast Example:

orange juice	1/2 cup
toast	1/2 slice
cereal, dry	3/4 cup
egg	1
milk, 2%	1/2 cup
margarine	1 tsp.

Lunch:
2 meat exchanges (list 5)

1-1/2 bread exchanges (list 4)

vegetable(s) as desired (list 1)
1 fruit exchange (list 3)
1/2 cup 2% milk (list 7)

Lunch Example:

cheese	2 1-oz. slices
beef bouillon	as desired
bread	1 slice
crackers, saltines	3 squares
tomato salad	as desired
apple	1 small
milk, 2%	1/2 cup
mustard	as desired

Dinner:
3 meat exchanges (list 5)
1 bread exchange (list 4)
vegetable(s) as desired (list 1)

1 vegetable exchange (list 2)
1 fruit exchange (list 3)
1 fat exchange (list 6)

Dinner Example:

chicken, baked	3 oz.
potatoes, mashed	1/2 cup
salad from list 1	
vegetables	as desired
peas	1/2 cup
fruit cocktail	1/2 cup
margarine	1 tsp.

Bedtime Feeding:
1 cup 2% milk (list 7)
or
1 fruit exchange (list 3)
1/2 bread exchange (list 4)

Bedtime Feeding Example:

milk, 2%	1 cup
or	
grapefruit juice	1/2 cup
graham cracker	1 square

Daily Menu Guide: 1500 Calories

Breakfast:
1 fruit exchange (list 3)
1-1/2 bread exchanges (list 4)

1 meat exchange (list 5)
2 fat exchanges (list 6)

1 cup 2% milk (list 7)

Lunch:
2 meat exchanges (list 5)
2 bread exchanges (list 4)
vegetable(s) as desired (list 1)
1 fruit exchange (list 3)
2 fat exchanges (list 6)

Dinner:
3 meat exchanges (list 5)
2 bread exchanges (list 4)

vegetable(s) as desired (list 1)

1 vegetable exchange (list 2)
1 fruit exchange (list 3)
2 fat exchanges (list 6)

Bedtime Feeding:
1 cup 2% milk (list 7)
1/2 bread exchange (list 4)
  or
1 meat exchange (list 5)
1 bread exchange (list 4)

Breakfast Example:

orange juice	1/2 cup
cereal, dry	3/4 cup
toast	1/2 slice
egg	1
bacon, crisp	1 slice
margarine	1 tsp.
milk, 2%	1 cup

Lunch Example:

cheese	2 1-oz. slices
bread	2 slices
tomato salad	as desired
apple	1 small
mayonnaise	2 tsp.

Dinner Example:

chicken, baked	3 oz.
potatoes, mashed	1/2 cup
bread	1 slice
salad from list 1 vegetables	as desired
peas	1/2 cup
fruit cocktail	1/2 cup
French dressing	1 tbsp.
margarine	1 tsp.

Bedtime Feeding Example:

milk, 2%	1 cup
graham cracker	1 square
or	
roast beef	1 oz.
bread	1 slice
mustard	as desired

Daily Menu Guide: 1800 Calories

Breakfast:	Breakfast Example:	
1 fruit exchange (list 3)	orange juice	1/2 cup
2 bread exchanges (list 4)	toast	2 slices
1 meat exchange (list 5)	egg	1
3 fat exchanges (list 6)	bacon, crisp	1 slice
	margarine	2 tsp.
1 cup 2% milk (list 7)	milk, 2%	1 cup

Lunch:	Lunch Example:	
3 meat exchanges (list 5)	cold cuts	2 1-1/2 oz. slices
	cheese	1 oz.
2 bread exchanges (list 4)	bread	2 slices
vegetable(s) as desired (list 1)	tomato salad	as desired
2 fruit exchanges (list 3)	apple	2 small
2 fat exchanges (list 6)	margarine	1 tsp.
	mayonnaise	1 tsp.

Dinner:	Dinner Example:	
3 meat exchanges (list 5)	chicken, baked	3 oz.
2-1/2 bread exchanges (list 4)	potatoes, mashed	1/2 cup
	bread	1-1/2 slices
vegetable(s) as desired (list 1)	salad from list 1	
	vegetables	as desired
1 vegetable exchange (list 2)	peas	1/2 cup
1 fruit exchange (list 3)	fruit cocktail	1/2 cup
2 fat exchanges (list 6)	margarine	2 tsp.

Bedtime Feeding:	Bedtime Feeding Example:	
1 cup 2% milk (list 7)	milk, 2%	1 cup
1 bread exchange (list 4)	graham crackers	2 squares
or	or	
2 bread exchanges (list 4)	bread	2 slices
1 meat exchange (list 5)	roast beef, lean	1 oz.
	mustard	as desired

Daily Menu Guide: 2000 Calories

Breakfast:
1 fruit exchange (list 3)
2-1/2 bread exchanges (list 4)

2 meat exchanges (list 5)
3 fat exchanges (list 6)

1 cup 2% milk (list 7)

Lunch:
3 meat exchanges (list 5)

3 bread exchanges (list 4)
vegetable(s) as desired (list 1)
1 fruit exchange (list 3)
2 fat exchanges (list 6)

Dinner:
3 meat exchanges (list 5)
3 bread exchanges (list 4)

vegetable(s) as desired (list 1)

1 vegetable exchange (list 2)
1 fruit exchange (list 3)
2 fat exchanges (list 6)

Bedtime Feeding:
1 cup 2% milk (list 7)
1 bread exchange (list 4)
  or
2 bread exchanges (list 4)
1 meat exchange (list 5)

Breakfast Example:
orange — 1
cereal, dry — 3/4 cup
toast — 1-1/2 slices
eggs — 2
bacon, crisp — 1 slice
margarine — 2 tsp.
milk, 2% — 1 cup

Lunch Example:
cold cuts — 2 1-1/2 oz. slices
cheese — 1 oz.
bread — 3 slices
tomato salad — as desired
apple — 1 small
margarine — 1 tsp.
mayonnaise — 1 tsp.

Dinner Example:
chicken, baked — 3 oz.
potatoes, mashed — 1/2 cup
bread — 2 slices
salad from list 1
  vegetables — as desired
peas — 1/2 cup
fruit cocktail — 1/2 cup
French dressing — 1 tbsp.
margarine — 1 tsp.

Bedtime Feeding Example:
milk, 2% — 1 cup
graham crackers — 2 squares
  or
bread — 2 slices
roast beef, lean — 1 oz.

Daily Menu Guide: 2500 Calories

Breakfast:
2 fruit exchanges (list 3)
3 bread exchanges (list 4)

2 meat exchanges (list 5)
3 fat exchanges (list 6)

1 cup 2% milk (list 7)

Breakfast Example:

orange juice	1 cup
cereal, dry	3/4 cup
toast	2 slices
eggs	2
bacon, crisp	1 slice
margarine	2 tsp.
milk, 2%	1 cup

Lunch:

3 meat exchanges (list 5)
4 bread exchanges (list 4)
2 fat exchanges (list 6)

vegetable(s) as desired (list 1)
1 fruit exchange
1 cup 2% milk (list 7)

Lunch Example:

cold cuts	2 1-1/2 oz. slices
mayonnaise	1 tsp.
bread	2 slices
cheese	1 oz.
mayonnaise	1 tsp.
bread	2 slices
dill pickle, radishes	as desired
apple	1 small
milk, 2%	1 cup

Dinner:
3 meat exchanges (list 5)
3 bread exchanges (list 4)

vegetable(s) as desired (list 1)

1 vegetable exchange (list 2)
2 fruit exchanges (list 3)
2 fat exchanges (list 6)
1 cup 2% milk (list 7)

Dinner Example:

chicken, baked	3 oz.
potatoes, mashed	1/2 cup
bread	2 slices
salad from list 1 vegetables	as desired
peas	1/2 cup
fruit cocktail	1 cup
butter	2 tsp.
milk, 2%	1 cup

Bedtime Feeding:
1 cup 2% milk (list 7)
2 bread exchanges (list 4)
1 meat exchange (list 5)
  or
2 bread exchanges (list 4)
1 meat exchange (list 5)
1 fat exchange (list 6)
1 fruit exchange (list 3)

Bedtime Feeding Example:

milk, 2%	1 cup
hamburger bun	1
roast beef	1 oz.
or	
hamburger bun	1
roast beef	1 oz.
mayonnaise	1 tsp.
grapefruit juice	1/2 cup

Daily Menu Guide: 3000 Calories

Breakfast:
1 fruit exchange (list 3)
3 bread exchanges (list 4)

2 meat exchanges (list 5)

4 fat exchanges (list 6)

1 cup 2% milk (list 7)

Midmorning Feeding:
1 cup 2% milk (list 7)
1 bread exchange (list 4)

Lunch:

3 meat exchanges (list 5)
3 bread exchanges (list 4)
3 fat exchanges (list 6)

vegetable(s) as desired (list 1)
1 fruit exchange (list 3)
1 cup 2% milk (list 7)

Midafternoon Feeding:
1 meat exchange (list 5)
2 bread exchanges (list 4)

Dinner:
3 meat exchanges (list 5)
2-1/2 bread exchanges (list 4)

vegetable(s) as desired (list 1)

1 vegetable exchange (list 2)
1 fruit exchange (list 3)
1 cup 2% milk (list 7)
3 fat exchanges (list 6)

Breakfast Example:

orange juice	1/2 cup
cereal, dry	3/4 cup
toast	2 slices
egg	1
ham	1 oz.
bacon, crisp	2 slices
margarine	2 tsp.
milk, 2%	1 cup

Midmorning Feeding Example:

milk, 2%	1 cup
graham crackers	2 squares

Lunch Example:

egg, hard-cooked and chopped	1
mayonnaise	2 tsp.
bread	1 slice
cold cuts	2 1-1/2 oz. slices
mayonnaise	1 tsp.
bread	2 slices
dill pickle, radishes	as desired
apple	1 small
milk, 2%	1 cup

Midafternoon Feeding Example:

cheese, American	1 oz.
bread	2 slices

Dinner Example:

chicken, baked	3 oz.
potatoes, mashed	1/2 cup
bread	1-1/2 slices
salad from list 1 vegetables	as desired
peas	1/2 cup
fruit cocktail	1/2 cup
milk, 2%	1 cup
margarine	3 tsp.

Bedtime Feeding:	Bedtime Feeding Example:	
1 meat exchange (list 5)	roast beef	1 oz.
2 bread exchanges (list 4)	hamburger bun	1
2 fat exchanges (list 6)	margarine	2 tsp.
"free" food as desired (list 1)	mustard	as desired
1 cup 2% milk (list 7)	milk, 2%	1 cup

—Courtesy of Eli Lilly and Company

Appendix E
Some Convenience Food Equivalents

RECOMMENDATIONS FOR PLACING CAMPBELL'S CONDENSED SOUPS INTO EXCHANGE LISTS

(These recommendations are based on a one cup portion when prepared according to directions on the label.)

Exchange substitution for
1-1/2 bread and 1 meat:
  Split Pea with Ham
Exchange substitution for
1-1/2 bread and 1/2 meat:
  Chili Beef
Exchange substitution for
1-1/4 bread and 1/2 fat:
  Tomato, Bisque of
Exchange substitution for
1 bread, 1 fat, and 1 vegetable B:
  Bean with Bacon
Exchange substitution for
1 bread, 1 vegetable B, and 1/2 meat
  Hot Dog Bean
Exchange substitution for
1 bread, 1/2 fat, and 1/4 vegetable B:
  Tomato Rice, Old Fashioned
Exchange substitution for
1 bread and 1/2 fat:
  Asparagus, Cream of
  Tomato
  Low Sodium Tomato*

Exchange substitution for
1 bread and 1/2 meat:
  Tomato-Beef Noodle-O's
Exchange substitution for
1/2 bread and 2 fat:
  Mushroom, Cream of
  Low Sodium Mushroom,
    Cream of*
Exchange substitution for
1/2 bread and 1 fat:
  Celery, Cream of
  Chicken, Cream of
  Mushroom, Golden
Exchange substitution for
1/2 bread, 1/2 fat, and
1/2 vegetable B:
  Clam Chowder Manhattan Style
  Golden Vegetable Noodle-O's
  Minestrone
Exchange substitution for
1/2 bread, 1/2 meat, and
1/2 milk:
  Clam Chowder, New England

146

Exchange substitution for
1/2 bread, 1/2 meat, 1/4 fat,
and 1/4 vegetable B:
   Noodles & Ground Beef
   Pepper Pot
Exchange substitution for
1/2 bread and 1/2 meat:
   Beef Noodle
   Curly Noodle with Chicken
   Turkey Noodle
   Low Sodium Turkey Noodle*
Exchange substitution for
1/2 bread, 1/2 milk, 1 fat, and
1/4 meat
   Shrimp, Cream of
Exchange substitution for
1/2 bread, 1/4 fat, 1/4 milk, and
1/4 vegetable B:
   Potato, Cream of
Exchange substitution for
1/2 bread and 1/4 meat:
   Chicken Gumbo
   Chicken Noodle
   Chicken Noodle-O's
   Chicken with Rice
   Chicken & Stars
Exchange substitution for
1 meat, 1/2 bread, and
1/2 vegetable B:
   Beef
Exchange substitution for
1/2 meat, 1/2 fat, and
1/4 bread:
   Chicken 'n Dumplings
Exchange substitution for
1/2 meat, 1/2 milk, and 1/4 bread:
   Oyster Stew

Exchange substitution for
1/2 meat and 1/2 vegetable B:
   Onion
Exchange substitution for
1/2 milk, 1 fat, and 1/4 bread:
   Cheddar Cheese
Exchange substitution for
2 vegetable B, 1/2 bread,
and 1/2 fat:
   Green Pea
   Low Sodium Green Pea*
Exchange substitution for
1 vegetable B, 1/2 bread,
and 1/2 fat:
   Black Bean
Exchange substitution for
1 vegetable B and 1/2 bread:
   Vegetable
   Low Sodium Vegetable*
   Vegetarian Vegetable
Exchange substitution for
1 vegetable B, 1/2 fat,
and 1/4 bread
   Chicken Vegetable
   Turkey Vegetable
Exchange substitution for
1 vegetable B and 1/2 fat:
   Vegetable, Old Fashioned
Exchange substitution for
1 vegetable B, 1/2 meat, and
1/4 bread:
   Scotch Broth
Exchange substitution for
1 vegetable B and 1/2 meat:
   Stockpot
   Vegetable Beef
   Low Sodium Vegetable Beef*

* Based on a one can portion Ready to Serve Low Sodium Soup.

Chunky Soups—Do Not Dilute (1 cup portion)

Exchange substitution for
1-1/2 bread, 1-1/2 meat, and
1 vegetable B:
   Chunky Split Pea with Ham
Exchange substitution for
1 bread, 1 meat, 1/2 fat, and
1/2 vegetable B:
   Chunky Sirloin Burger
Exchange substitution for
1 bread, 1 vegetable B, and
1/2 meat:
   Chunky Clam Chowder
Exchange substitution for
1-1/2 meat, 1 vegetable B, and
1/2 bread:
   Chunky Chicken with Rice

Exchange substitution for
1-1/4 meat, 1 bread, and
1/2 vegetable B:
   Chunky Beef
Exchange substitution for
1-1/4 meat and 1 bread:
   Chunky Chicken
Exchange substitution for
1 meat, 1/2 bread, and
1/2 vegetable B:
   Chunky Turkey
Exchange substitution for
1 vegetable B, 1/2 bread, and
1/2 fat
   Chunky Vegetable

Recommendations for Placing Other Campbell Products into Exchange Lists

Campbell's Canned Products (1/2 cup portion)

Exchange substitution for
1-1/2 bread, 1 vegetable B, and
1/2 fat:
   Home Style Pork & Beans
Exchange substitution for
1-1/2 bread and 1/2 meat:
   Pork & Beans with
   Tomato Sauce
Exchange substitution for
1-1/4 bread, 1 vegetable B, and
1/2 fat:
   Beans & Franks in Tomato &
   Molasses Sauce

Exchange substitution for
1-1/4 bread, 1 vegetable B, and
1/2 fat:
   Barbecue Beans
   Old Fashioned Beans in
      Molasses and Brown Sugar
      Sauce
Exchange substitution for
1 bread and 1 meat:
   Beans 'n Beef in Tomato Sauce

Swanson Canned Products (1 cup portion)

Exchange substitution for
2 meat and 1-1/2 bread:
   Chili Con Carne with Beans
Exchange substitution for
2 meat, 1 vegetable B, and
1/2 bread:
   Beef Stew
Exchange substitution for
1-1/4 meat, 1 vegetable B, and
1/2 bread:
   Chicken Stew

(1/2 cup portion)

Exchange substitution for
1 meat, 1/2 bread, and 1/2 fat:
   Chicken a la King

(1/2 cup portion)

Exchange substitution for
1 meat and 1/2 bread:
   Creamed Chipped Beef

Franco-American Canned Products (1 cup portion)

Exchange substitution for
2 bread, 1 vegetable B,
and 1/4 fat:
   Spaghetti in Tomato Sauce
      with Cheese
Exchange substitution for
2 bread, 1/2 fat, and
1/4 vegetable B:
   Italian Style Spaghetti in
      Tomato-Cheese Sauce
   "SpaghettiOs" in Tomato and
      Cheese Sauce
Exchange substitution for
1-1/2 bread, 1-1/4 meat, 1 fat,
and 1/2 vegetable B:
   Spaghetti 'n Beef in
      Tomato Sauce
   Spaghetti with Meatballs in
      Tomato Sauce

Exchange substitution for
1-1/2 bread, 1-1/4 meat, and
1 fat:
   Macaroni 'n Beef in Tomato Sauce
   "SpaghettiOs" with Sliced Franks
      in Tomato Sauce
Exchange substitution for
1-1/2 bread, 1-1/2 vegetable B,
and 1-1/4 meat:
   Beef Raviolios in Meat Sauce
Exchange substitution for
1-1/2 bread, 1/2 fat, and
1/2 milk:
   Macaroni & Cheese
Exchange substitution for
1-1/4 bread, 1-1/4 meat, 1/2 fat,
and 1/4 vegetable B:
   "SpaghettiOs" with Little
      Meatballs in Tomato Sauce

Swanson Brand Frozen
Prepared Products

Individual Meat Pies
(8 ounces each)

Exchange substitution for
3 bread, 4 fat, 1 meat, and
1 vegetable B:
 Chicken Pie
Exchange substitution for
2-1/4 bread, 4 fat, 1 meat, and
1 vegetable B:
 Turkey Pie
Exchange substitution for
2 bread, 3 fat, 1-1/2 meat, and
1 vegetable B:
 Beef Pie

Deep Dish Meat Pies
(16 ounces each)

Exchange substitution for
3 bread, 5 fat, 3 meat, and
2 vegetable B:
 Chicken Pie
Exchange substitution for
3 meat, 3 fat, 2-1/2 bread, and
2 vegetable B:
 Beef Pie
 Turkey Pie

TV Brand Entrees
(1 complete entree)

Exchange substitution for
3 meat, 2 bread, and 1-1/2 fat:
 Fried Chicken with Whipped
 Potatoes
Exchange substitution for
2 meat, 2 bread, and
1-1/2 fat:
 Salisbury Steak with
 Crinkle-Cut Potatoes
Exchange substitution for
2 meat, 1-1/2 fat, 1 bread, and
1 vegetable B:
 Meat Loaf with Tomato Sauce and
 Whipped Potatoes

Exchange substitution for
2 meat, 2 bread, and 1/4 fat:
 Turkey • Gravy • Dressing with Whipped
 Potatoes
Exchange substitution for
2 meat, 1-1/2 bread, 1-1/2 fat, and
1/2 vegetable B:
 Meatballs with Brown Gravy
 and Whipped Potatoes
Exchange substitution for
2 meat, 1-1/2 bread, 1/2 fat, and
1/4 vegetable B:
 Breaded Veal with Spaghetti
 in Tomato Sauce

One half cup portion of any of the following may be used without counting as part of a meal plan:

Beef Broth (Bouillon)	Tomato Juice
Consommé (Beef) gelatin added	"V-8" Cocktail Vegetable Juice

These recommendations have been developed by Campbell Soup Company, based on the Standard Exchange Units set forth by the American Dietetic Association, American Diabetes Association, and Public Health Service Department of Health, Education and Welfare.

—Courtesy of Campbell Soup Company

Appendix F
U S V Ethnic Diets

(Recommended Foods to Eat Each Day)

Food Exchange List	Units Daily	
Milk	2 glasses	Choose skim milk. You may use 1/4 cup of powdered skim milk.
Vegetable	1 serving	Choose a 1/2 cup serving of one of the following: beets, carrots, onions, peas or turnips. You may use a combination to make a 1/2 cup serving.
Fruit	3 servings	Select only fruits that are fresh, frozen or canned without sugar added. Choose as one serving one of the following: 1 orange or 1/2 grapefruit or 1/2 cup of juice, 1 apple, peach or pear, 2 plums, 1 cup of berries, 12 grapes, 1/4 cantaloupe, 1/2 banana, 2 prunes or 2 dried figs.
Bread	6 servings	Choose as one serving one of the following: 1 slice of bread or 1/2 cup of cereal, 1/2 cup of rice, 1/2 cup of pasta, or 1/2 cup of lima, kidney or navy beans, or chick peas, or 1 potato. You may have a double serving of one food but count it as two servings. For example, 1 cup of spaghetti is two servings.
Meat	6 ounces	Choose beef, lamb, pork, veal, chicken, turkey, or fish. These are 3-ounce servings:

1 slice of roast beef   2 small meatballs
1 small serving of fish   1 chicken leg

1 egg, 1/4 cup of cottage cheese, 1 slice of cheese or luncheon meat, or 1/4 cup of canned fish is about a 1-ounce meat serving.

Fat   4 servings Choose as one serving one of the following: 1 small pat of butter or margarine, 1 teaspoonful of olive or cooking oil, 1 tablespoonful of cream cheese, 5 small olives or 1 slice of bacon.

"No Count" Foods Eat these foods as desired, but in moderation: red or green peppers, mushrooms, tomatoes, cauliflower, celery, cucumbers, fennel, green beans, salad greens—chicory, escarole, chard, spinach, asparagus, broccoli, eggplant, zucchini and pickles; clear broth, coffee and tea.

Season foods with: herbs, spices, garlic, lemon, and vinegar.

Do Not Eat These Foods Sugar and syrups, honey, jams and jellies, sweetened fruits and beverages, pies, cakes, pastries, sweet desserts, and candy.

Sample Menu for One Day

Breakfast:

orange juice—1/2 cup
cheese—1 slice
bread—1 slice, margarine—1 pat
milk—1/2 glass
coffee

Lunch:

pasta—1 cup with 1 meatball and tomato sauce
green salad, lemon
milk—1/2 glass
apple—1
coffee or tea

Dinner:

vegetable soup with carrots and beans
fish—3 ounces
salad of sliced tomatoes and marinated mushrooms
bread—1 slice, margarine—1 pat
grapes—12
tea

Evening Snack:

milk—1 glass
bread—1 slice, margarine—1 pat

JEWISH DIABETIC DIET

(Recommended Foods to Eat Each Day)

Food Exchange List	Units Daily	
Milk	2 glasses	Choose skim milk or buttermilk made with skim milk. You may use 1/4 cup of powdered skim milk or 1 cup of plain yogurt.
Vegetable	1 serving	Choose a 1/2 cup serving of one of the following: beets or borscht (without sugar), carrots, onions, scallions, green peas, squash, or turnips. You may use a combination to make a 1/2 cup serving.
Fruit	3 servings	Select only fruits that are fresh, frozen, or canned without sugar added. Choose as one serving one of the following: 1 orange, tangerine or 1/2 grapefruit or 1/2 cup of juice, 1 apple, pear, peach or 2 apricots or 2 plums, 1/2 cup of applesauce, 1/2 banana, 1/4 cantaloupe, 1 cup of watermelon, 1 cup of berries, 2 dried prunes or apricots, 1/4 cup of prune juice, 2 tablespoons of raisins or 12 grapes.
Bread	6 servings	Choose as one serving one of the following: 1 slice of challah, rye, or pumpernickel bread, 1 small roll or bagel, 1/2 piece of matzo, 1/2 cup of rice, noodles, cooked barley, or kasha (buckwheat groats), 1/2 cup of cooked cereal, 1/2 cup of cooked split peas, chick peas, lima beans, navy beans, or lentils, 1 small potato, 1

small corn on the cob, 3 tablespoons of farfel, 2 tablespoons of matzo meal or 3 soda crackers.

Meat   **6 ounces**   Choose beef, lamb, liver, veal, chicken, turkey, or fish. These are 3-ounce servings:

2 small lamb chops	1 small fish (flounder)
1 small piece of beef liver	1 chicken leg

1 egg, 1/4 cup of cottage, pot or farmer cheese, 1/4 cup of canned tuna or salmon, 3 medium sardines or 2 tablespoonfuls of peanut butter is about a 1-ounce meat serving. You may also use 1 frankfurter or 1 ounce of gefilte fish, herring, smoked white fish, salmon, cooked pastrami, or corned beef as part of the meat serving.

Fat   **4 servings**   Choose as one serving one of the following: 1 small pat of butter or margarine, 1 tablespoon of cream cheese, 2 tablespoons of sour cream, 1 teaspoonful of oil or chicken fat or 6 small nuts.

"No Count" Foods   Eat these foods as desired, but in moderation: asparagus, broccoli, cabbage, sauerkraut, cauliflower, celery, cucumbers, eggplant, mushrooms, green or wax beans, red or green peppers, escarole, lettuce, radishes, spinach, parsley, tomatoes, sour or dill pickles.

Season foods with herbs, spices, garlic, lemon, and vinegar. You may use horseradish, cranberries, cinnamon, ginger, nutmeg, mint, dry mustard and paprika, coffee and tea.

Do Not Eat These Foods   **Sugar and syrups, honey, molasses, jams and jellies, pies, cakes, cookies, pastries, candy, sweetened soft drinks, sweetened fruits, and beverages.**

Sample Menu for One Day

Breakfast:

grapefruit—1/2
bagel—1
cream cheese—1 tablespoon
smoked salmon—1 ounce (small slice)
milk—1/2 glass
coffee

Lunch:

borscht—1/2 cup
sour cream—2 tablespoons
sliced egg—1
cottage cheese—1/4 cup
tomato and lettuce
bread—2 slices, margarine—1 pat
stewed prunes—2
milk—1/2 glass
coffee or tea

Dinner:

roast chicken—3 ounces
baked noodle pudding—
    1/2 cup noodles, 1 teaspoon fat
green beans
marinated cucumbers
challah—1 slice
applesauce—1/2 cup
tea and lemon

Evening Snack:

plain yogurt—1 cup or
    1 glass buttermilk
soda crackers—3

MEXICAN-AMERICAN DIABETIC DIET

(Recommended Foods to Eat Each Day)

Food Exchange List	Units Daily	
Milk	2 glasses	Choose skim milk. You may use 1/4 cup of powdered skim milk.
Vegetable	1 serving	Choose a 1/2 cup serving of one of the following: carrots, peas, onions, pumpkin, beets, or squash. You may use a combination to make a 1/2 cup serving.
Fruit	3 servings	Select only fruits that are fresh, frozen, or canned without sugar added. Choose as one serving one of the following: 1 orange or 1/2 grapefruit or 1/2 cup juice, 1 apple, pear, peach, or guava, 2 apricots, 1/2 small mango, 1/3 papaya, 1/2 cup of fresh pineapple or 2 slices of canned pineapple, 1/4 cantaloupe, 2 fresh figs or 2 tablespoonfuls of raisins.
Bread	6 servings	Choose as one serving one of the following: 1 slice of bread or 1 roll, 1 tortilla, 2-1/2 tablespoonfuls of flour or cornmeal, 1/2 cup of rice or beans (frijoles), 1/2 cup of cooked cereal, hominy or spaghetti, 1 small corn on the cob or 1 small white potato or 1 small sweet potato or yam.

Meat	6 ounces	Choose beef, pork, lamb, veal, chicken, turkey, or fish. These are 3-ounce servings:

    2 very small pieces   2 small meatballs
      of chicken
    1 pork chop   1 small piece of fish
1 egg, 1/4 cup of cottage cheese, 1 slice of cheese or luncheon meat, 1 frankfurter, 1 (5x2-inch) piece of tripe, 1/4 cup canned fish, or 2 tablespoonfuls of peanut butter is about a 1-ounce meat serving.

Fat   **4 servings**   Choose as one serving one of the following: 1 small pat of butter or margarine, 1 teaspoonful of oil or lard, 1 teaspoonful of mayonnaise, 1/8 avocado, 1 slice of crisp bacon, 6 small nuts or 5 small olives. Be sure to count the fat used to cook foods.

"No Count" Foods   Eat these foods as desired, but in moderation: asparagus, broccoli, Brussels sprouts, cabbage, cauliflower, celery, cucumbers, lettuce, cacti leaves (nopales), mushrooms, green beans, green and red peppers, tomatoes, spinach and salad greens such as kale, mustard or beet greens, chard and collard, radishes, and pimiento.

You may have coffee, tea, clear broth or bouillon, unsweetened gelatin, and sour pickles. Season foods with herbs, spices, garlic, lemon, and vinegar. You may use cinnamon, celery and garlic salt, paprika, cayenne, mustard, mint, parsley, and vanilla.

Do Not Eat These Foods   Sugar and syrups, honey, jams and jellies, desserts with sugar, cakes, cookies, pastries, candy, sweetened condensed milk, sweetened soft drinks, sweetened fruits and beverages.

Sample Menu for One Day

Breakfast:
orange juice—1/2 cup
egg—1
fried potatoes—1/2 cup
tortilla—1 or 1 slice dry toast
skim milk—1/2 glass
coffee

Lunch:
vegetable soup with meat
refried beans—1/2 cup with
   1 slice cheese
green salad with lemon
tortilla—1
apricots—2
skim milk—1/2 glass
coffee or tea

Dinner:
fried chicken—2 small pieces
rice with tomatoes and spice—1/2 cup
cooked carrots—1/2 cup
apple—1
coffee or tea

Evening Snack:
taco made with meat, chicken or
   cheese—1
skim milk—1 glass

SOUTHERN AMERICAN "SOUL" DIABETIC DIET

(Recommended Foods to Eat Each Day)

Food Exchange List	Units Daily	
Milk	2 glasses	Choose skim milk or buttermilk made with skim milk. You may use 1/4 cup of powdered skim milk or 1 cup of plain yogurt.
Vegetable	1 serving	Choose a 1/2 cup serving of one of the following: beets, onions, pumpkin, winter squash, green peas, rutabagas or turnips, or carrots. You may use a combination to make a 1/2 cup serving.
Fruit	3 servings	Select only fruits that are fresh, frozen, or canned without sugar added. Choose as one serving one of the following: 1 orange or 1/2 grapefruit or 1/2 cup juice, 1 apple, pear, peach or 2 apricots, 1/2 cup of fresh pineapple or 2 slices of canned pineapple, 1 cup of watermelon, 1/4 cantaloupe, 1/2 banana, 1 cup of berries, 2 prunes, 1/4 cup of prune juice, or 12 grapes.
Bread	6 servings	Choose as one serving one of the following: 1 slice of bread or 1 biscuit or 1 muffin or 1 cube (1-1/2 inch) of cornbread, 2-1/2 tablespoonfuls of flour or cornmeal, 1/2 cup of cooked cereal, hominy grits or rice, 3/4 cup of dry cereal, 1/2 cup of spaghetti, macaroni or noodles, or 1/2 cup of cooked beans (lima, kidney, pinto or

butter beans), 1/2 cup of cooked split or black-eyed peas, 1/3 cup of corn, I small corn on the cob, 1 cup of popcorn, 2/3 cup of parsnips, 1/4 cup of sweet potato or yam, 1 small white potato or 2 graham crackers.

Meat	6 ounces	Choose beef, lamb, pork, ham, liver, veal, chicken, turkey, duck, or fish. These are 3-ounce servings:

    1 pork chop   1 small piece of fish
    2 very small pieces   1 small piece of
       of baked chicken   of round steak

1 egg, 1 slice of cheese or luncheon meat, 1/4 cup of cottage cheese or canned tuna or salmon, 1 frankfurter, 1 piece (5x2-inch) of tripe, or 2 tablespoons of peanut butter is about a 1-ounce meat serving.

Fat   **4 servings**   Choose as one serving one of the following: 1 small pat of butter or margarine, 1 slice of crisp bacon, 1 teaspoonful of oil or lard, 1 teaspoonful of mayonnaise or 6 small nuts. Be sure to count the fat used to cook foods.

"No Count" Foods   Eat these foods as desired, but in moderation: asparagus, broccoli, cabbage, celery, cucumbers, green beans, red and green peppers, tomatoes, spinach, greens such as collard, dandelion, mustard, beet, carrot tops, kale, and poke, chicory, escarole, parsley, okra, eggplant, and rhubarb. You may have coffee, tea, clear broth or bouillon. Season foods with herbs, spices, garlic, lemon, and vinegar.

**Do Not Eat
These Foods**   **Sugar and syrups, honey, molasses, jams and jellies, sweetened condensed milk, pies, cakes, cookies, pastries, candy, candy-coated gum, sweetened soft drinks, sweetened fruits and beverages.**

Sample Menu for One Day

Breakfast:
orange juice—1/2 cup
grits—1/2 cup
egg—1
crisp bacon—1 slice
milk—1 glass
coffee

Lunch:
kidney beans (1/2 cup) with onions and
    pepper—1 teaspoon oil and vinegar
collard greens with ham (2 ounces)
bread—1 slice, margarine—1 pat
peach—1
coffee

Dinner:
baked round steak—3 ounces
tomatoes and okra
rice—1/2 cup
*turnips—1/2 cup
*biscuit—1
apple—1
coffee

Evening snack:
cornbread
buttermilk—1 glass

*1 teaspoon lard in cooking turnips or
1 pat margarine with the biscuit

PUERTO RICAN DIABETIC DIET

(Recommended Foods to Eat Each Day)

Food Exchange List	Units Daily	
Milk	2 glasses	Choose skim milk. You may use 1/4 cup of powdered skim milk.
Vegetable	1 serving	Choose a 1/2 cup serving of one of the following: beets, carrots, onions, peas, pumpkin, squash, or turnips. You can use a combination to make a 1/2 cup serving.
Fruit	3 servings	Choose as one serving one of the following: 1 orange or 1/2 grapefruit or 1/2 cup of juice, 1 apple or pear, peach or guava, 1/2 small mango, 1/3 papaya, 1/2 cup of fresh pineapple or 2 slices of canned unsweetened pineapple, 1/2 banana, 1 cup of watermelon or 10 West Indian cherries (acerolas).
Bread	6 servings	Choose as one serving one of the following: 1 slice of bread or 1 roll or 1/2 cup of cereal or 1/2 cup of rice or 1/2 cup of macaroni or 2-1/2 tablespoonfuls of flour or cornmeal or 1/2 cup of beans (these may be cow peas [frijoles], chick peas [garbanzos], kidney beans [habichuelas coloradas], lima beans [habos], navy beans [habichuelas blancas] or pigeon beans [grandules]) or 1 small corn on the cob, 1/4 green plantain, 1 small white potato, 1/4 cup of sweet potato, 1 small tanniers or 1 small breadfruit.

Meat	6 ounces	Choose beef, lamb, pork, liver, veal, chicken, turkey or fish. These are 3-ounce servings:
		  3 small pieces of pork 2 small meatballs
		  1 small serving of fish 1 chicken leg
		1 egg, 1/4 cup of cottage cheese, 1 slice of cheese or luncheon meat, 1/4 cup of canned fish, or 2 tablespoonfuls of peanut butter is about a 1-ounce meat serving.

Fat	4 servings	Choose as one serving one of the following: 1 small pat of butter or margarine, 1 teaspoonful of oil or cooking fat, 1 tablespoon of cream cheese, 1/8 avocado, 6 small nuts, 5 small olives, or 1 teaspoonful of prepared anchiotespice.
"No Count" Foods		Eat these foods as desired, but in moderation: cabbage, celery, cucumber, eggplant, chayote, cauliflower, red and green peppers, green beans, tomatoes, pimiento, ensalada—chicory, escarole, collard greens (berza), lettuce, mustard greens, spinach, pickles; clear broth, coffee and tea. Season foods with herbs, spices, garlic, lemon and vinegar. You may use cinnamon, ginger, anise seed, parsley, sesame seed, marjoram, sweet chili pepper (aji dulce), paprika, cayenne, and coriander.
Do Not Eat These Foods		**Sugar and syrups, honey, molasses, jams and jellies, pies, cakes, cookies, pastries, candy, sweetened condensed milk, sweetened soft drinks, sweetened fruits and beverages.**

Sample Menu for One Day

Breakfast:
orange—1 medium (or 10 acerolas)
egg—1 soft-cooked
hard roll, margarine—1 pat
milk—1 glass
coffee

Lunch:
asopao of 1/2 cup of rice and
    1/2 cup of beans and seasonings
luncheon meat—2 slices
ensalada—green salad with garlic and lemon
avocado—1/8
papaya—1/3 medium (or 1 apple)
coffee

Dinner:
baked fish—3 ounces
vegetable stew (sancocho)—green peppers,
    1/2 cup pumpkin, 1 potato
bread—1 slice, margarine—1 pat
pineapple—1/2 cup
coffee

Evening snack:
milk—1 glass
plantain or potato chips—1/2 cup

CHINESE DIABETIC DIET

(Recommended Foods to Eat Each Day)

Food Exchange List	Units Daily	
Milk	2 glasses	Choose soybean milk (tou fu chiang) or cow's milk. You may use 1/4 cup of powdered skim milk.
Vegetable	1 serving	Choose a 1/2 cup serving of one of the following: beets, carrots, onions, pumpkin, rutabagas, turnips, scallions, green peas, snow peas, squash or bamboo shoots. You can use a combination to make a 1/2 cup serving.
Fruit	3 servings	Choose as one serving one of the following: 1 orange or 1/2 grapefruit or 1/2 cup of juice, 1 apple, pear, peach or 2 fresh apricots, 1/4 cantaloupe, 1/2 small mango or 1/8 honeydew melon, or 1/2 cup of fresh pineapple or 2 slices of canned unsweetened pineapple, 1 cup of berries, 1 cup of watermelon, 10 litchi nuts, 2 dried figs, or 1/2 banana.
Bread	6 servings	Choose as one serving one of the following: 1/2 cup of cooked rice or 1/2 cup of cooked cereal, macaroni or noodles, 1 slice of Chinese or regular bread, 1 roll, 1/2 cup of dried beans (black beans), or peas, 1/4 cup of soybeans, 1 white potato, 5 saltine crackers, or 2 tablespoons of cornstarch (in cooking).

Meat	6 ounces	Choose beef, lamb, pork, liver, veal, chicken, turkey, or fish. These are 3-ounce servings:

2 small pieces of chicken
3 small pieces of pork
1 small serving of fish
5 small shrimp, 1 egg, bean curd

1 egg, 1 slice of cheese or luncheon meat, 1/4 cup of canned fish, or 2 tablespoonfuls of peanut butter is about a 1-ounce meat serving. You may use 1 ounce of bean curd (tou fu lao) or eel (huang shan) or octopus or squid as part of the meat serving.

Fat 4 servings Choose as one serving one of the following: 1 small pat of butter or margarine or 1 teaspoonful of cooking oil such as soybean, sesame, peanut or corn oil, 1 slice of crisp bacon or 6 small nuts.

"No Count" Foods Eat these foods as desired, but in moderation: asparagus, broccoli, cabbage, celery cabbage, Chinese cabbage (bok choy), cauliflower, celery, cucumber, eggplant, escarole, lettuce, tomato mushrooms, red and green peppers, radishes, spinach, green beans, bean sprouts (hsiang chun ya), and greens such as beet, chard, collard, kale, turnip, and mustard (gai choy) greens, Chinese parsley (chi tsai), and zucchini.

Season foods with herbs, spices, garlic, lemon, and vinegar. You may use monosodium glutamate, soy sauce, ginger, anise seeds, szechwan pepper.

Do Not Eat These Foods Sugar and syrups, honey, jams and jellies, sweetened fruits and beverages, cakes, cookies, pastries, candy and seasonings and sauces with sugar such as ketchup, chili sauce, and plum sauce.

Sample Menu for One Day

Breakfast:
orange—1 medium
cooked oatmeal—1/2 cup
steamed Chinese bread—1 slice,
    margarine—1 pat
soybean milk—1 glass
tea

Lunch:
clear soup with 1 ounce bean curd
    and 1/2 cup noodles
roast pork—2 small pieces with bamboo
    shoots or carrots—1/2 cup of "no count"
    vegetables—1 teaspoonful of oil
cooked rice—1/2 cup
apple—1
tea

Dinner:
chicken—3 ounces with bean sprouts,
    cabbage, ginger and 1 teaspoonful of oil
spinach and garlic
cooked rice—1/2 cup
litchi nuts—10 or 1/4 cantaloupe
tea

Evening snack:
soybean milk—1 glass
saltine crackers—5, margarine—1 pat

—Courtesy of USV Pharmaceutical Corp.,
Tuckahoe, N.Y. 10707

Appendix G

Special Ethnic Exchange List of the
Diabetes Association of Southern California

Special Exchange Lists for Latin American Foods

1 thin corn tortilla	1 bread
1 thin flour tortilla	1 bread and 1 fat
2 tamales	1 bread and 1 fat
1 enchilada	1 bread and 1 fat

Arroz con Carne (rice with meat):

1 cup of rice	2 bread
2 ounces of ground meat	2 meat
1 teaspoon of fat	1 fat

Fidello con Carne (vermicelli with meat):

1 cup of vermicelli	2 bread
2 ounces of ground meat	2 meat
1 teaspoon of fat	1 fat

Papas con Carne (potatoes with meat):

1 small potato	1 bread
2 ounces of ground meat	2 meat
1 teaspoon of fat	1 fat

Refried Beans:

1/2 cup of cooked beans	1 bread
1 teaspoon of fat	1 fat

Chicharo con Carne (peas with meat):

1/2 cup of cooked peas	1 vegetable (list 2-B)
2 ounces of ground meat	2 meat
1 teaspoon of fat	1 fat

Chili con Carne:

1/4 cup pinto beans	1/2 bread
4 teaspoons of flour	1/2 bread
1 teaspoon of fat	1 fat
2 ounces of ground meat	2 meat
tomato sauce	1/2 cup (count as vegetable from list 2-A)

1 tortilla de maíz	1 cambio de pan
1 tortilla de harina	1 cambio de pan y 1 cambio de grasa
2 tamales	1 cambio de pan y 1 cambio de carne
1 enchilada	1 cambio de pan y 1 cambio de carne

Arroz con Carne:

1 taza de arroz	2 cambios de pan
2 onzas de carne picada	2 cambios de carne
1 cucharita de grasa	1 cambio de grasa

Fideo con Carne:

1 taza de fideo	2 cambios de pan
2 onzas de carne picada	2 cambios de carne
1 cucharita de grasa	1 cambio de grasa

Papas con Carne:

1 papa pequena	1 cambio de pan
2 onzas de carne picada	2 cambios de carne
1 cucharita de grasa	1 cambio de grasa

Frijol Refrito:
1/2 taza de frijol, cocido
1 cucharita de grasa

Chicharo con Carne:
1/2 taza de chicharo cocido
2 onzas de carne picada
1 cucharita de grasa

Chile con Carne:
1/2 taza de frijo pinto
4 cucharitas de harina
1 cucharita de grasa
2 onzas de carne picada
salsa de tomate

1 cambio de pan
1 cambio de grasa

1 cambio de vegetal
(lista 2-B)
2 cambios de carne
1 cambio de grasa

1/2 cambio de pan
1/2 cambio de pan
1 cambio de pan
2 cambios de carne
1/2 taza (úselo como
un vegetal de
lista 2-A)

Chinese Menu

Exchanges are listed for the following foods to help you when eating out. (Courtesy of *House of Kwong* menu.)

Appetizers:

Rumaki
spiced chicken livers and water chestnuts, wrapped in crisp bacon.
2 pieces = 1 meat + 1 fat

Shiu Mi
minced water chestnuts, chives, and pork, wrapped in thin noodle paste then steamed.
2 pieces = 1/2 bread + 1/2 meat

Entrees (best to stick with simple items):

Chow Lung Har
fresh lobster tails cooked in a delicately flavored garlic sauce
1 order = 3 meat + 1 fat

Fung Gawn Har
shrimp, chicken liver, imported mushrooms, cooked together in rich chicken broth
1 order = 3 meat + 2 fat

Mun Yee Mein
braised noodles, topped with breast of chicken, mushrooms, bamboo shoots, water chestnuts and chinese peas
1 order = 2 bread + 2 meat + 1 fat

Seasonal vegetables and beef
1 cup = 1-1/2 meat + A vegetables

Tso See Gau
shredded lettuce, chicken, rice noodles, green onions, tossed with tantalizing sauce
1 order = 2 meat + 1-1/2 bread + 1 fat

Miscellaneous:

Egg Flower Soup	broth with egg
	1 cup = 1/2 meat
Won Ton Soup	broth with won ton added, green onion
	1 cup = 1/2 bread + 1/2 meat (2 won ton)
Fried Rice	rice, pork *or* shrimp, green onion, egg
	1 cup + 1-1/2 bread + 1/2 meat + 1 fat
Fortune Cookies	2 cookies = 1 bread
Egg Roll	2" section of roll = 1 bread + 1 B vegetable
Chicken Chow Mein	
	1 cup + 1 meat + 1/2 bread

Avoid the following:

barbecued ribs
fried shrimp
almond cakes
candied ginger + coconut
fried won ton
foods cooked in oyster sauce

Mexican Menu

Exchanges (approximate) are listed for the following foods to help you when eating out. (Courtesy of *El Torito* menu.)

Salads:
  Ensalada Compuesta
                   mixed green salad
                   1 serving = free (ask for dressing on side, if
                   desired, 1 tablespoon = 1 fat)
  Ensalada de Aguacate
                   sliced avocado, diced tomatoes on bed of
                   lettuce (be careful here) 1 serving without
                   dressing = 3 fat + A vegetables

Entrees:
  Omelet de Queso   cheese omelet, rice, and beans
                    1 order = 4 meat + 2 bread + 2 fat
  Chile Verde   diced pork simmered with green chile, rice or
                    beans
                    1 order = 3 meat + 1 bread + 2 fat
  Pollo en Mole   breasts of chicken cooked in a rich Mexican
                    sauce, served with rice
                    1 order = 3 meat + 1-1/2 bread + 2 fat
  Arroz con Camaron Guaymas shrimp simmered in a spicy sauce and
                    served with Mexican rice
                    1 order = 3 meat + 1-1/2 bread + 2 fat
  Chile con Carne with Beans
                    pinto beans, ground beef, chili sauce
                    1 cup = 1 meat + 3 bread + 2 fat (average)

Exchange List for McDonald's

1 plain hamburger	=	1 meat 2 bread
1 cheeseburger	=	1-1/2 meat 2 bread
1 Big Mac	=	2-1/2 meat 3 bread 1 fat
1 Quarter Pounder	=	3 meat 2 bread
1 Quarter Pounder with cheese	=	4 meat 2 bread
6 French fries (1/2"x1/2"x2")	=	1 bread 1 fat
1/2 chocolate shake	=	1/2 milk 1 bread (an estimate) 2 fat

—Courtesy of Pam Fulkerson, registered dietician,
Northridge Hospital, Northridge, California

Appendix H

Chart of the More Common Foreign
Equivalents for Oral Drugs Sold in the
United States

Oral Drugs

Orinase—Tolbutamide		Tolinase—Tolazamide		DBI—Phenformin	
Rastinon	Europe	Orabetta	Chile	Insural	Latin
Artosin	Europe	Tolisan	Denmark		America
Dolitol	France		Iceland	Inural	
Mobenol	Canada	Norglycin	Germany	Retards	Latin
Rastinon	Canada	Tolanase	England		America
Orinase	Canada		Canada	Dibotin	United
Diabin	Japan				Kingdom
Mellitus D	Japan			Insural	New
Yosulant	Mexico				Zealand
Oralin	Philippines				Australia
Orsinon	Israel			Dibein	Scandinavia

Glucophage—Metformin:* France, 1/20 to 1/30 the strength of Phenformin.

Silubin—Buformin:* Germany, Australia, Switzerland, and countries behind the Iron Curtain, 1/2 the strength of Phenformin.

*Strengths may vary. Consult your doctor before leaving.

Diabenese—Chlorpropamide		Dymelor—Acetohexamide	
Catanil	Italy	Dimelin	Japan
Chloronase	Germany	Dimelor	England
Chlorodiabet	Spain	Ordimel	Norway,
Diabetoral	Germany		Netherlands,
Mellinese	Denmark		Sweden, and Chile

—Courtesy of Squibb

Appendix I

Counting Carbohydrates in Foreign Countries

Foreign Foods and Their Equivalents

Spain: Paella is rice, and 1/3 cup of rice is equal to one slice of bread. Paella is fine in moderation, but bread and other starchy food must then be omitted.

Israel: Peta, though unleavened, is bread, just as matzo is starch. This must be considered with dining native.

Germany: An eight ounce drink of ale equals 1-1/2 slices of bread.

Scotland and England: Porridge is like boiled oatmeal and three ounces equals ten grams of carbohydrates. Puddings, such as Yorkshire, tarts, pies, and tapioca may prove too rich for a diabetic diet.

Europe: Since a continental breakfast may be only a roll and coffee, it may be wise to order two breakfasts.

Jamaica: Fruits are delicious, but beware. One half a mango equals one half small banana or a small orange.

Mexico: Tortilla chips are equal to one gram of carbohydrate.

Japan: Sukiyaki, made with questionably amounts of sugar and/or sweet wine should be excluded. Tempura should be eaten with the batter coating counting as a bread exchange. Mizutaki (beef or chicken chunks cooked in broth) or sashimi (raw fish) are fine.

France: A little dry wine will not upset the glucose tolerance. Acceptable wines in France and elsewhere containing 1.2% or less grams of sugar in a 3-1/3 ounce serving are listed below:

Bordeaux	Burgundy	Chablis
Vin ordinaire	Average	Dry champagne
Claret	Australian	Hock (English term
California claret	Beaunè	for Rhine wine)
Graves	Californian	Moselle
Dry sauterne	Pommard	

Other permissible drinks:
Absinthe
Brandy
Akvavit—one ounce
Kummel—one ounce
Dry sherry—three ounces

But say NO to:
lemonades
nondiabetic tonic water
ginger beer
stout
cider
Port
sweet wines

In Ireland, Scotland, and the U.S., scotch, rye, vodka, and bourbon are permissible *in moderation*. Remember that hypoglycemia and intoxication can be—and are—often confused.

Weights and Measures:
1 gram = .03 oz. 10 gram = .35 oz. (1/3 oz.) 1 liter = 1.057 qt.
To change grams to ounces, divide by 30. To change ounces to grams or cc, multiply by 30.

—Courtesy of Squibb

Appendix J

Some Helpful Tips on Filling Your Insulin Syringe

Fourteen Helpful Tips

1. Separate tabs and peel apart to open package.

2. Remove syringe/needle unit from package.

3. Before removing needle guard push needle guard with twisting action to tightly secure needle to syringe.

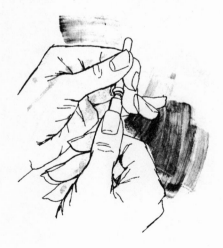

4. Remove needle guard by pulling straight off. Do not twist when removing.

5. Check label of insulin vial for any special instructions. Do not shake vial. Agitate gently.

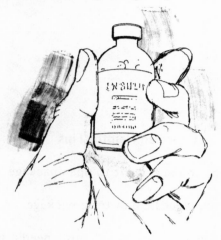

6. Clean rubber stopper of insulin vial by swabbing with alcohol soaked cotton (or pre-packaged disposable alcohol swabs).

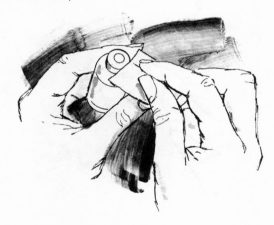

7. Pull plunger of syringe back to roughly the same number of units of insulin you use.

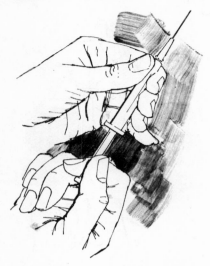

8. Insert needle straight through vial stopper and inject this air into the vial.

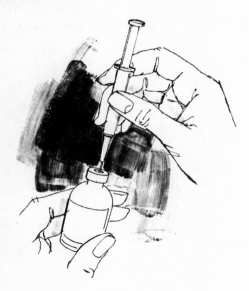

9. Turn vial upside down.

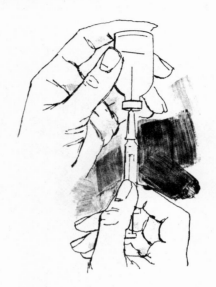

10. Make certain that the point of the needle inside the vial is well under the surface level of the insulin.

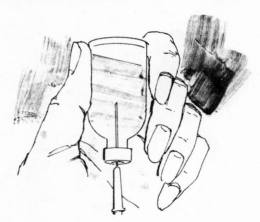

11. While holding the syringe and vial vertically with the point upwards, withdraw the plunger so that the front rib line registers one or two units more than you will inject.

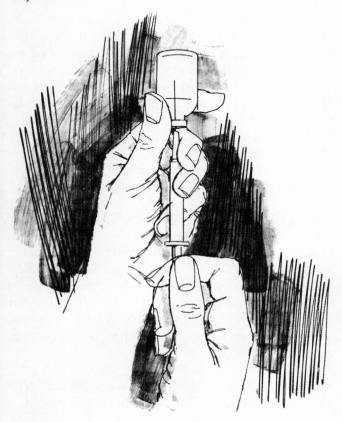

12. If a bubble (or bubbles) is entrapped in the insulin, a sharp tap with your finger against the barrel of the syringe will usually release it. If the syringe is held vertically, the bubble will rise into the tip of the syringe. Expel the excess amount of insulin back into the vial so that you end up with the exact number of units you take.

Air bubbles per se are not dangerous for your type of injection except as they affect the correct measurement of your insulin dosage. They occur because of the air space in the cannula (or shaft) of the needle and the air space in the tip of the syringe which precedes the insulin into the syringe when you withdraw it from the vial. When they occur, they are usually entrapped by the sterile inert medical grade silicone that is used on the plunger tip to make disposable syringes work smoothly and easily. Usually larger bubbles can be easily dislodged and removed by the procedure suggested above. Very tiny bubbles are of little concern since they would be the last thing expelled from the syringe and would displace only the small amount of insulin that would normally be left in the needle cannula.

13. Note: If you use two types of insulin, your doctor may recommend that you proceed as follows. Into the first vial of insulin, inject an amount of air equal to the amount of that insulin to be used. Now inject an appropriate amount of air into the other vial of insulin and withdraw the proper amount of insulin. Reinsert needle into the first insulin vial, withdraw prescribed amount and mix the two insulins in the syringe by gentle agitation.

14. Withdraw syringe and needle from the vial. You are now ready to proceed with your injection.

—Courtesy of Becton Dickinson

Appendix K

Two Accepted Techniques for Self-Injection

INSULIN INJECTION TECHNIQUE

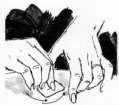

1. With thumb and index finger of one hand, stretch the skin away from clean area selected for injection and cleanse area with an alcohol swab. Using a circular motion, wipe injection area from the center out toward the edge of injection site.

3. Release pressure on skin and use freed hand to hold syringe while other hand pulls back slightly on plunger.

If blood appears in bottom of syringe barrel, pull unit out of skin slightly — 1/16 to 1/8 inch — to remove needle tip from blood vessel. Pull back slightly on plunger again. If more blood appears, select new injection site. Replace the needle if you do this because the first one is contaminated.

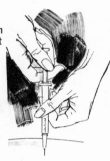

2. Keeping skin stretched, grasp syringe firmly near its tip with other hand, taking care not to touch sterile needle.

Quickly thrust needle straight into injection site, as illustrated. Thrust needle in up to its hub.

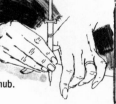

ALTERNATE METHOD TO STEP 2.

2a. If injection is to be made into an area with only a thin layer of fat, pinch a fold of skin between fingers, rather than stretching skin. This will keep needle from penetrating into a muscle.

Taking care not to touch sterile needle, grasp syringe firmly near its tip.

Quickly thrust needle straight into injection site, as illustrated. Thrust needle in up to its hub.

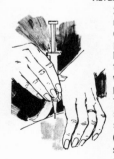

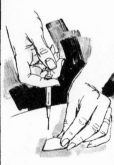

4. Slowly push plunger all the way down to inject insulin.

5. Hold alcohol swab close to needle hub. withdraw syringe and attached needle rapidly, in a straight line.

6. As needle comes out of skin, quickly place alcohol swab over injection site.

7. Briefly apply firm pressure on alcohol wipe over injection site.

8. Record injection site and do not use it again for at least 14 days.

INSULIN INJECTION INTO THE ARM
This technique utilizes the hand as a self-injector
for entering arm injection sites at approximately a 90° angle.

After preparing injection site:

1. Hold syringe over cleaned injection site of opposite arm between thumb and index finger, as illustrated.

2. Place outer edge of hand on arm, below cleaned injection area. Palm of hand will be facing away from arm as you look toward injection site.

3. With outer edge of hand, press down on arm to stretch skin slightly in injection area.

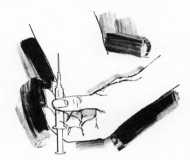

4. Grasping syringe firmly, thrust needle into skin by flipping wrist quickly toward the arm, while outer edge of hand is still applying pressure. Release pressure and raise hand slightly from arm once needle is inserted.

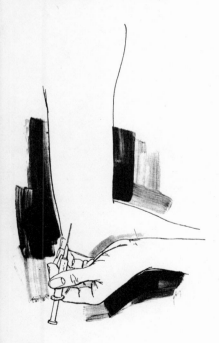

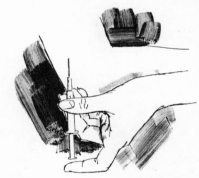

5. Holding syringe barrel steady, replace index finger with third finger.

Position fingers high enough up on barrel so that freed index finger can be used to:

a. Push plunger up slightly to check for blood in barrel. (Select new injection site if blood appears. Use a new sterile needle, because the first one is now contaminated.)

b. Depress plunger slowly to inject insulin.

6. Withdraw syringe and needle rapidly in a straight line and briefly apply firm pressure to injection site with clean alcohol swab.

—Courtesy of Becton Dickinson

Appendix L

What Foods Can Be Served on Diabetic Diets

This list is not a diet. It gives only general information about the kinds of foods that may be served on the diet prescribed for a diabetic.

	Foods Allowed	Foods to Avoid
Meat, Fish Poultry	All kinds served plain or in combination with allowed foods. Visible fats should be removed.	Fried meat, except when fat allowance used for frying. All dipped in batter or crumbs.
Milk	Whole milk, skim, or buttermilk, pasteurized, homogenized, evaporated, dried, or concentrated.	Chocolate or other sweetened milks. Sweetened condensed milk.
Cheese	All kinds	None
Eggs	Prepared any way without fat	Fried or scrambled eggs, unless part of the fat allowance is used for cooking.
Fruits	All fresh, canned, or frozen.	Any canned or frozen with sugar added. Check labels.

	Allowed	Not Allowed
Vegetables	All fresh, canned or frozen. Raw or cooked. Vegetables may be combined with sugar-free gelatin.	None
Cereals and Bread	Whole grain, or enriched breads and cereals, macaroni, noodles, rice, spaghetti.	Sugar coated cereals. Any bread or rolls to which sugar or frosting have been added.
Fats, Oils	All, including mayonnaise and French dressing made without sugar.	Thickened gravies, unless made from allowed flour and fat. Sweetened mayonnaise or oil dressing.
Soups	Soups made from allowed foods. Canned soups may be substituted for allowed foods. (See Exchange Lists.)	None, if made from allowed foods or if substitutions made. (See Exchange Lists.)
Sweets	None	All forms—jams, jelly, preserves, honey, syrup, molasses, candy.
Desserts	Fruit may be served plain or in combination with sugar-free gelatin. Baked custards made from egg and milk allowance and sweetened with saccharin or other artificial sweetener.	All pastries, cakes, sweetened desserts. Desserts made of flavored gelatin sweetened with sugar. Plain sponge cake and ice cream may be used occasionally. (See Bread Exchange List.)
Beverages	Milk or juices as allowed. Coffee, tea (beverage may be sweetened with saccharin or other artificial sweetener).	Milk drinks or carbonated beverages sweetened with sugars or syrups.

Condiments   All spices and seasonings. Mustards, ketchup,   Any seasonings or sauces containing sugar. Any
                horseradish, sour pickles, unsweetened dill   pickles made with sugar.
                pickles, vinegar, lemon.

—*Courtesy of the Diabetes Association*
of Southern California